Scaling Effective School Mental Health Interventions and Practices

Lee Kern • Mark D. Weist
Samuel D. McQuillin
Editors

Scaling Effective School Mental Health Interventions and Practices

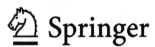

Editors
Lee Kern
Department of Education
and Human Services
Lehigh University
Bethlehem, PA, USA

Mark D. Weist
Department of Psychology
University of South Carolina
Columbia, SC, USA

Samuel D. McQuillin
Department of Psychology
University of South Carolina
Columbia, SC, USA

ISBN 978-3-031-68167-7   ISBN 978-3-031-68168-4   (eBook)
https://doi.org/10.1007/978-3-031-68168-4

This Springer imprint is published by the registered company Springer Nature Switzerland AG
The registered company address is: Gewerbestrasse 11, 6330 Cham, Switzerland

If disposing of this product, please recycle the paper.

This book is dedicated to Alexa. Your insight and compassion amaze me. I cherish every minute with you.

Mom

I am dedicating this book to my "second mom," Dixie, with thanks for your love, prayers, and support over the years.

Mark

To my beloved wife, Melissa, and our wonderful children, Molly, Kate, and Walker. Your love and joy inspire me every day.

Sam

Preface

In this book, we address the goal of scaling effective school mental health (SMH) practices and interventions for children and youth. As readers are keenly aware, we edited this book in the context of a global mental health crisis for all people, but especially for children and youth, which is characterized by unprecedented distress and a widening supply and demand gap between the number of trained providers and the ability to meet wide ranging social, emotional, behavioral, and mental health needs of young people. Supported by strong evidence, schools are the most critical youth serving system to promote positive mental health, well-being, and academic success of students, with countless barriers to access to effective programming reduced or removed.

We emphasize the importance of expanding access to mental health practices and interventions, while also maintaining effectiveness of this programming in complex and changing systems. Yet these two elements, scale and effectiveness, can often feel at odds with each other. Efforts to scale services often come at the expense of fidelity and efforts to maximize the fidelity of implementation often lack scalability. We hold that several advances in the field have reduced this tension between scalability and effectiveness, and we share information on these advances. As editors of this book, we invited authors who have successfully unpacked aspects of this conundrum and have addressed these dual elements in service of promoting equitable and effective services for children and youth.

This book advances scholarship in this area in three important ways. First, we synthesize modern literature on tiered support systems (e.g., multitiered systems of support) with a particular emphasis on interdisciplinary collaboration in the context of significant workforce challenges. Second, we highlight several innovations in intervention, screening, training, and collaboration that emphasize both scale and effectiveness. Third, we have edited this book to include practical guidance for realizing these concepts in the real-world environment of schools, characterized by a range of diverse programming; sometimes effective, and unfortunately, in many cases not so.

We hope educational leaders, teachers, policy makers, allied health and mental health staff, community partners, and researchers find this text useful in understanding modern scientific research on scaling effective school mental health. We believe readers will also find value in the practical applications of this research that have high significance for effective practice and advances in policy.

If our society is to realize a more equitable, effective, and robust child and youth mental health infrastructure, it will require expanded collaboration, innovation, and systems-level changes. We hope that this book provides a path forward in each of these domains. Combined, the three of us have more than 70 years of experience in this field, and we hope that ideas and strategies found in this book lead to the overall improvement and broad scaling up of effective SMH programs within schools, school districts, states, and regions, building from the foundation of effective vertical (e.g., states to districts to schools) and horizontal (e.g., interdisciplinary teamwork in a school building) collaboration informed by and guided by diverse community partners, especially the students and families served by these programs.

Bethlehem, PA, USA   Lee Kern

Columbia, SC, USA   Mark D. Weist

Columbia, SC, USA   Samuel D. McQuillin

Contents

Chapter 1
Key Themes for Scaling Effective School Mental Health Programs

Mark D. Weist, Samuel D. McQuillin, and Lee Kern

1.1 Building an Effective Multitiered System of Support

The foundation for the work described in this book is well-functioning multitiered systems of support (MTSS) in schools. This reflects the public health prevention framework that was later matched to the work of schools, as detailed in Chap. 2 (this volume). MTSS includes Tier 1 programming for all students (e.g., climate enhancement, universal prevention strategies); Tier 2 early intervention programming (e.g., skills training groups, mentoring programs, classroom-based support) for some students, such as those contending with conditions of risk or showing early signs of problems; and Tier 3 more intensive and individualized intervention programming (e.g., cognitive behavioral therapy for students presenting with depression and/or anxiety) for students showing clear evidence of more serious concerns (e.g., established mental health diagnoses). In our view, MTSS is best articulated by the Positive Behavioral Interventions and Supports (PBIS) framework, widely implemented in nearly 30,000 schools in the United States (see www.pbis.org). As modeled by schools implementing PBIS, effective MTSS includes the core practices of resource mapping and needs assessment; assuring strong, inclusive, and well-functioning teams; enabling broader constituent involvement; and elevating the voice and leadership of students and families. Other important core practices include choosing, implementing, and refining evidence-based practices (EBPs) within and across tiers; effective data-based decision-making, including screening for social, emotional, behavioral, and mental health (SEBMH) concerns; and connecting

M. D. Weist (✉) · S. D. McQuillin
University of South Carolina, Columbia, SC, USA
e-mail: weist@mailbox.sc.edu; mcquills@mailbox.sc.edu

L. Kern
Lehigh University, Bethlehem, PA, USA
e-mail: lek6@lehigh.edu

© The Author(s), under exclusive license to Springer Nature Switzerland AG 2024   1
L. Kern et al. (eds.), *Scaling Effective School Mental Health Interventions and Practices*,
https://doi.org/10.1007/978-3-031-68168-4_1

students to appropriate more intensive supports at Tiers 2 and 3. Additional critical emphases include focusing on equity to assure effective supports for youth of color; monitoring the fidelity of implementation and making adjustments accordingly; assessing intervention impacts on students; engaging in continuous quality improvement; promoting effective vertical and horizontal collaboration; and addressing workforce challenges including building emphases on task shifting. We elaborate on each of these themes below.

1.2 Resource Mapping and Needs Assessment

Resource mapping and needs assessment, fully described in Chap. 4 (this volume), is a process that is important at multiple levels of scale, including school building, district, and state levels. At each of these levels, the process should focus on understanding the following aspects of programming: what is being implemented, if it addresses clearly identified needs, whether it is being implemented with fidelity, and whether it is having intended positive effects on students' SEBMH functioning. The National Center on PBIS (see www.pbis.org) has three tools that can assist in assessing the nature of programming, with an emphasis on fidelity (i.e., whether interventions are implemented as designed). At the school level, the Tiered Fidelity Inventory (TFI) can be used for these purposes. The TFI is a reliable and valid measure that assesses the extent to which school staff are implementing core features of PBIS overall and at each individual tiers (see https://www.pbis.org/resource/tfi). Please note a TFI 3.0 version is in development by the PBIS center, and should be available for use later in 2024. The TFI should be completed by teams responsible for MTSS implementation in schools, in this case the lead team for SEBMH, with the measure completed at the beginning of the school year to identify areas to strengthen programming. It can then be completed at the end of the academic year to assess progress, or on a yearly schedule at the beginning of the school year.

Fidelity at the district level can be assessed using the District Systems Fidelity Inventory (DSFI). The PBIS Center states the purpose of the DSFI "is to guide District Leadership Teams in the assessment, development, and execution of action plans that promote the capacity for sustainable, culturally and contextually relevant, and high-fidelity implementation of multi-tiered social, emotional, and behavioral systems of support and practices. The DSFI and process were designed to guide initial action planning, progress monitoring and annual evaluation of fidelity of implementation and impact" (see https://www.pbis.org/resource/dsfi). Kittelman et al. (2023) evaluated the DSFI and found that it measured nine aspects of district systems: leadership, stakeholder engagement, funding and alignment, policy, workforce capacity, training, coaching, evaluation, and local implementation demonstrations.

At the state level, the State Systems Fidelity Inventory (SSFI) can be used to assess implementation. According to the PBIS Center, the SSFI "is designed to assist State Leadership Teams and similar organizational units with (a) initial assessments of the extent to which there is the capacity to implement PBIS; (b) action planning to guide resource allocation during the process of PBIS implementation; and (c) periodic assessments of the capacity of a state or region to sustain PBIS implementation and expansion" (see https://www.pbis.org/resource/ssfi).

Another more informal and interactive approach for resource mapping is to present the triangle (see Chap. 2, this volume) reflecting the MTSS with Tiers 1, 2, and 3, and have staff list programming occurring at each tier, and then evaluate whether the programming is working, along with successes and challenges experienced and ideas for overcoming challenges. Again, this more informal analysis can be conducted at school, district, and state levels. Through use of the formal measures mentioned (TFI, DSFI, SSFI) and this more informal interactive approach, additional analyses should be conducted related to financial and other resources (e.g., staff time) being used to implement the various programs. Analyses should determine whether these resources are adequate and, if not, how they could be enhanced. Notably, this resource mapping process will often reveal that programming is not being implemented as intended, not having the predicted positive impacts, or even having negative impacts. This points to the importance of systematically de-implementing or sunsetting programs that are not working. This latter process can be challenging if a school, district, or state has invested significant resources in a program that is not working (e.g., the cognitive dissonance experienced by leaders when expensive programs are not being implemented and/or appear ineffective).

Ideally occurring together with resource mapping is systematic needs assessment, again conducted at school building, district, and state levels. This can be accomplished through quantitative analyses, such as reviewing building- and district-level data on school climate, student discipline referrals, inequities in discipline referrals for students of color, student/family receipt of indicated Tier 2 and Tier 3 programming, inequities in service receipt, and measures of students' academic progression (e.g., patterns of matriculation and graduation, standardized test scores). Similarly, state-level data can be used to compare indicators across school districts, and to compare performance of states within a region (e.g., comparing data for North and South Carolina, identifying strengths and challenges of each, and building collaboration between the two states to share lessons learned on enhancing strengths and overcoming challenges). In this regard, communities of practice are very helpful in building systems of collaboration, establishing mutual support, and sharing lessons learned (see Chap. 3, this volume). As above, these quantitative data can be paired with qualitative data, such as focus group themes and key informant interviews with the diverse staff and constituent groups invested in school mental health (SMH), including education, mental health, and other youth-serving system leaders and staff (e.g., child welfare, juvenile justice, primary care), advocacy organizations, family and youth leaders, researchers, and government officials.

1.3 Effective Teams

The MTSS is the foundation for effective programming in SMH, and within MTSS, the functioning of teams is likely the most important quality indicator of overall MTSS functioning. Unfortunately, the common picture in schools is the presence of numerous teams, most not functioning well, with inconsistent scheduling, limited attendance, poorly formulated agendas, and a lack of action planning with consistent follow-up on team-identified actions across the MTSS. At the school building level, an important process is to map all teams within a school (e.g., PBIS team, Crisis Team, Student Assistant Team, and Special Education–Focused Teams) and identify one team to be strengthened to coordinate assessment and plans focused on improving student SEBMH functioning (see Eber et al., 2020). This team should be inclusive of the right staff and disciplines, including school administrators, SMH providers (school- and community-employed), educators, allied health staff (e.g., nursing, speech, and occupational therapy), and families and youth. The Team Initiated Problem Solving (TIPS; Chaparro et al., 2022) approach is the most commonly used strategy to organize the work of teams, ensuring they are inclusive of the right members, meet consistently, use organized agendas, keep ongoing meeting notes, develop and implement action strategies, and track the impact of action strategies on the fidelity of implementation of EBPs along with their impact on important student outcomes through progress monitoring (e.g., student attendance, academic engagement, grades, discipline encounters). More information on effective teams can be found in a comprehensive monograph of this theme developed by the National PBIS Center (Splett et al., 2024).

At the district level, it is important to develop a strong leadership team that coordinates state to district to building support, and in turn, tracks what is happening in school buildings to identify and disseminate positive lessons learned and best practices. Here, the Interconnected Systems Framework (ISF) for PBIS and SMH (see Barrett et al., 2013; Eber et al., 2020) is highly informative. The ISF describes strategies to promote well-functioning MTSS in schools, amplified by strong partnerships (and memoranda of agreement, MOA) between schools and community mental health agencies to enable a seamless system of augmented programming across all tiers, with community mental health staff viewed and acting as if they are employees of the school. This involves community staff being involved to some extent in Tier 1 and Tier 2 programming, and strengthening evidence-based Tier 3 programming. In this context, a strong District-Community Leadership Team (DCLT), including education and mental health leaders, and leaders from other youth serving systems (as above), along with advocates and family/youth leaders, systematically guides the work occurring in all school buildings, drawing from and directing state-level and other resources (e.g., from federal grants, foundation funded initiatives) to support the work in buildings, and in turn, tracking what is happening in buildings and disseminating best practices out to other buildings. A promising strategy is for DCLTs to support model demonstration projects (MDPs) where particular buildings implement strong MTSS with EBPs across tiers (with coaching support). The MDP documents and disseminates their experiences to enable uptake and scaling to other buildings. Similarly, a state-level DCLT can coordinate programming across school districts, using MDPs of district level initiatives to promote dissemination and scaling of best practices.

A critical challenge in the United States for scaling effective practices within school districts and buildings is associated with federalism, or states' rights and local control. These practices are compounded by site-based management of schools, resulting in a hodgepodge of programming within and across school districts (see Weist et al., 2009). The resulting extreme variability creates barriers to communication and collaboration, as there are many different approaches to assessment and intervention, and lack of formal strategies for discussion and improvement across levels of scale. Here, there is a need for standardization of evidence-based measurement and intervention approaches, which facilitates communication and collaboration, and standardized reporting of progress at district and state levels.

1.4 Enhancing Family and Student Leadership

A very significant challenge in SMH is the prevailing pattern of limited youth and family voice and leadership in programming of the schools' MTSS. This is cogently summarized by Hart's (1994) ladder, which presents an 8-point continuum of youth voice, with low numbers (say 1–3) reflecting adult-centric environments in which staff guide all programming and tell students what to do. Instead, schools' MTSS should be co-created by educators, collaborating mental health staff, and youth and families. Truly co-created environments result in higher scores on Hart's ladder (e.g., scores of 6–8). Notably, our experience is that schools often recognize the importance of student and family leadership in programming, but do little to eventuate this strategy. In fact, we commonly find resistance to family involvement in the work of schools, and meetings that are characterized by criticizing and blaming of families, versus viewing and treating them as key collaborators. With support of the National PBIS Center, an e-book on changing the paradigm toward more significant family and youth leadership was published (Weist et al., 2017) and widely disseminated. A second edition of this e-book is in progress, and the Family-School-Community Alliance (see https://fscalliance.org) is actively working to improve research, practice, and policy relevant to family and youth leadership in schools.

1.5   Selecting and Installing Evidence-Based Practices Across Tiers

Choosing, installing, and refining EBPs across tiers is an essential practice at school building and district levels (see Chap. 2, this volume). At the building level, the lead SEBMH team should focus first on universal programming for all students at Tier 1. Such programming includes efforts to scan and improve the school environment (e.g., identifying times of day and places associated with higher discipline problems and initiating corrective measures) and to put in place school-wide programming for all students. There is a range of universal prevention programs that can be implemented at these tiers with a number of relevant repositories, such as the What Works Clearinghouse of the U.S. Department of Education (https://ies.ed.gov/ncee/wwc/), and programs endorsed by the Collaborative for Academic, Social, and Emotional Learning (CASEL, see www.casel.org). Additional interventions, programs, and procedures are detailed in Chap. 2 (this volume).

At Tier 2, effective programming often includes mentoring support (e.g., Check In Check Out; Hawken et al., 2014), support for teachers for effective classroom management (see Kern et al., 2016), skill training groups (https://www.pbis.org/pbis/tier-2), and providing brief focused mental health support to students and their families (see Lyon et al., 2015). At Tier 3, school- and community-employed mental health staff should be engaged in practices that have strong empirical support. In addition, a functional behavioral assessment (FBA) is critical for identifying environmental events associated with emotional and behavioral problems that can be addressed with intervention. Chapter 2 (this volume) provides a thorough description of interventions at Tiers 2 and 3.

Across tiers, there is a need for ongoing fidelity monitoring to assure that practices are being delivered as intended, and progress monitoring to document positive impacts or lack of responsiveness occurring within the school and for students/families. As presented earlier, when programs are not delivered as intended and/or not having positive impacts, active consideration should be placed on de-implementing or sunsetting them.

An important issue to consider for programming delivered across all tiers is proprietary programs marketed to schools that have mixed, poor, or no evidence base for effectiveness (see George et al., 2013). Efforts by private companies to market programs to schools are significant. This can create stress and cognitive dissonance for school leaders who purchase expensive programs that are not working (i.e., being reluctant to abandon them related to funds that have been allocated). Notably, there are many effective programs that are in the public domain and available to schools at no cost or at cost.

As presented earlier, a key function at the district level is to coordinate EBPs delivered in individual school buildings. Unfortunately, there is often a lack of guidance and ongoing coaching of common EBPs by districts to buildings, leaving implementation decisions to individual schools related to site-based management. This again leads to extreme variability in programming across schools and presents significant limitations to centralized district support for schools to implement EBPs. Instead, there should be an emphasis on standardization in empirically supported assessment and intervention strategies across schools. As above, ideally there is a well-functioning DCLT inclusive of the right leadership, coordinating implementation of common EBPs across schools through strong coaching support, sharing lessons learned, building mutual support among schools, and developing school-level MDPs that serve as exemplars for other schools.

1.6   Using Data for Decision-Making

The collection of student data in schools throughout the United States has accelerated in the past few decades, spurred by No Child Left Behind legislation (Daly et al., 2006). With justification, educators regularly lament the voluminous number of tests they must administer. Among their many concerns is that data often are not shared with those positioned to make changes in response to areas of need. In addition, data frequently are not portrayed in a format that allows for easy interpretation and are insufficiently granular to assist educators with important decision-making. Hence, for data to be useful in the process of data scaling SMH, they must be purposeful and strategic.

SMH data are particularly important in the context of MTSS for a number of reasons. The primary reason is that, apart from externalizing problems (e.g., aggression, disruption), educators are not especially adept at identifying students experiencing mental health concerns, particularly internalizing concerns (e.g., depression, anxiety, trauma-related) and problems frequently are not detected until symptoms become severe (von der Embse et al., 2018; Weist et al., 2018). This issue is exacerbated as students enter middle and high school where they rotate from class to class, typically spending a limited amount of time with each teacher and personal interactions may be scarce. Compounding this problem is the many mental health concerns that emerge around adolescence. Thus, objective data are needed to identify students with mental health needs. Such data should be collected with the deliberate purpose of establishing thresholds to determine those students who will receive mental health support.

A second benefit of data is that they can be used to match student needs to potentially effective interventions. This is the case for both determining intervention intensity (e.g., Tier 2, Tier 3) and the type of intervention students will receive (e.g., anxiety, social skills, trauma). Using data to match student needs to intervention a priori avoids implementation of ineffective interventions, delay in providing effective intervention, and possibly an increase in problem intensity. This is significant when considering the limited number of minutes in a school day, rendering time afforded for mental health intervention nominal.

A third reason data-based decision-making is crucial pertains to measuring intervention effectiveness. Data are needed to draw conclusions about whether an intervention is working. Interventions that are not sufficiently effective can be modified by making common and evidence-based adaptations (e.g., Kern et al., 2020; Majeika et al., 2020), such as increasing their intensity (e.g., frequency). Alternatively, absent any suggestion of effectiveness, an intervention can be substituted with another.

1.7   Screening for Student SEBMH Concerns

Data-based decision-making also points to the very important role of systematic screening for students' SEBMH concerns, which continues to occur in a limited fashion in schools. Barriers related to poor infrastructure for such screening, schools' inexperience in the same, and reticence to screen for problems that cannot be addressed due to schools' limitations in mental health capacity have hampered wide-scale implementation (Weist et al., 2007). Traditionally, schools have used observation to screen for students' SEBMH concerns, such as identifying students with failing grades, discipline problems, or excessive absences. However, these observational methods will fail to detect many students in need. In one study (Splett et al., 2018), observational methods identified only about 10% of students with these concerns. When adding a systematic screener identification increased to over 30%, and notably about half of these additionally identified students had serious concerns (often internalizing problems) that were not being addressed. Building policy and practice support for such screening should emphasize that mental health conditions represent serious barriers to learning for students, and that without systematic screening there will be many students who flounder academically. Collecting screening data can also be used for advocacy with district, state, and other policy leaders to increase SMH providers in schools (Weist et al., 2007).

However, and as is emphasized in Chap. 5 (this volume), with the expansion and increased accessibility of instruments suited to school use, screening for students' SEBMH problems is fortunately increasing. Importantly, valid and reliable screening instruments have been developed that demand little teacher time (Oakes et al., 2017). Although screening measures can identify significant social, emotional, and behavioral problems, they also detect emerging problems, providing educators the opportunity to intervene early, before student challenges become intensive. Early intervention promises resolution of problems before they significantly interfere with a student's academic progress, social and developmental functioning, and overall wellbeing. Further, the need for intensive interventions that require substantial resources to address serious student concerns is reduced.

Data from SEBMH screening measures are best interpreted in conjunction with other school-collected data. For instance, information about school attendance or office disciplinary referrals can supplement screening information, informing school teams about how mental health challenges manifest relative to student functioning and the potential of intervention effectiveness. For example, student with anxiety who is frequently absent is unlikely to fully benefit from an anxiety program delivered only during the school day. Similarly, academic performance data helps educators understand the extent to which emotional and behavioral problems are hindering academic progress, allowing the team to assess the need for supplemental academic supports.

As detailed in Chap. 5, (this volume), there are an increasing number of SEBMH screening systems available to schools. Historically, many of these measures have been expensive, and as mentioned, schools often lack infrastructure and resources to conduct such screening effectively. With the move toward less expensive measures, improvements in infrastructure, and documentation of the benefits of screening on student and staff functioning, SEBMH screening is becoming more common. Based on our experiences with schools and districts across the country, the status of the screening remains somewhat limited, but progress is encouraging, as such screening should be viewed as a lynchpin for effective and scaled SMH programming.

1.8 Effectively Employing Data to Identify and Monitor Tier 2 and Tier 3 Supports/Interventions

As schools undertake the resource mapping process (Chap. 4, this volume), the availability of interventions at each tier becomes clear. As the full complement of tiered supports is developed, school screening data become meaningful and useful to the extent they are linked to available supports. To assure screening data are directly linked to interventions, schools must first summarize the data. This involves designating a person to download, organize, and summarize data in a meaningful fashion that allows for easy interpretation (see Chap. 5, this volume, for an example). The next undertaking is to aggregate the screening data with other available school data to fully inform each student's intervention needs. Schools should establish cut-off risk scores on screeners that will align with the level (e.g., Tier 2, Tier 3) and type (e.g., social skills group) of intervention indicated. Examples of additional school data to simultaneously consider are academic progress, which indicates whether there is a need for supplemental academic support, and office disciplinary referrals, which often suggest the location and characteristics of behavioral problems, narrowing suitable intervention options.

After students are connected to appropriate interventions, their progress is evaluated on a regular basis (see Chap. 2, this volume). This allows school teams to determine whether an intervention is effective and should be maintained, faded, or discontinued or whether insufficient progress indicates the intervention should be substituted with an alternative or additional interventions added. To make these decisions, flexible criteria should be established a priori. Decision criteria are especially important for tiered systems of support, where students should seamlessly move across (and within) tiers.

1.9   Focusing on Equity to Assure Appropriate Supports for Students of Color

There is a strong and growing literature base documenting that youth of color disproportionally experience school discipline as well as exclusion from needed supports and services (e.g., Bal et al., 2019; Tefera & Fischman, 2020). Efforts to improve equity for these youth should include assessment and intervention practices. In terms of assessment, the SEBMH lead team, in their ongoing data-based decision-making, should view and analyze data that are disaggregated for students' gender and race/ethnicity with emphasis on student discipline data, screening data, and connection of students to Tier 2 and Tier 3 supports. Discipline data include office referrals for behavioral problems, in-school suspensions, out-of-school suspensions, and expulsions. Commonly, these data will identify disparities, with youth of color often receiving more of each of these exclusionary discipline practices. McIntosh et al. (2018) underscored the importance of identifying vulnerable decision points; that is, using school data connected to contexts and time periods to identify when and which types of students are more likely to receive school discipline. For example, these data may show that discipline is more likely to happen when there are large groups of students congregating in an area of the building before lunch time, or in particularly before larger events like assemblies, and that during these time periods, Black students (especially Black males) are more likely to be disciplined (McNeill et al., 2016). These analyses should then lead to training of staff on this pattern of inequity, along with measures to reduce the likelihood of contexts-in-time increasing the likelihood of discipline events. Here, "neutralizing routines" can be used to counter the impact of vulnerable decision points; for example, training staff on unconscious bias that operates for all people (Benson & Fiarman, 2020), and having staff pause and reflect, before responding in situations that have been clearly identified as vulnerable decision points.

Reflecting themes of discipline and programming inequity, we documented, through a randomized controlled trial in elementary schools in two southeastern communities, that the Interconnected Systems Framework (ISF, strong school-mental health connections and focus on all core MTSS practices), as compared to PBIS and typical co-located mental health programming, was associated with overall reductions in student discipline, reduced discipline for youth of color, and increased likelihood of Tier 2 and Tier 3 support for youth of color (Weist et al., 2022a). These improvements were related to the ISF's emphasis on improved team functioning and data-based decision-making, including ongoing training and coaching on discipline-related inequities and ways to prevent them.

1.10 Monitoring and Improving the Fidelity of Implementation

Interventions should be deemed ineffective when students show no signs of improvement in targeted areas. It may be the case, however, that student data indicate no improvement because the intervention was not implemented as it was designed. This common problem can be due to the lack of competence in providers, implementation drift (i.e., gradual changes in the way intervention is implemented over time), inadequate capacity, or simply forgetting. Evidence-based interventions are so considered because they have been experimentally tested, which involves articulating the specific components anticipated to be critical for behavior change along with parameters of implementation, such as dosage (e.g., how many sessions or hours students must receive for expected impact). For an intervention to be potentially effective, it must have been implemented in the in the way it was proposed and tested. Hence, there should confidence that interventionists are implementing interventions as designed, also known as fidelity of implementation or intervention integrity. Only after interventions have been implemented with integrity can decisions be made about effectiveness.

The importance of fidelity of implementation cannot be understated. Students must receive potentially effective interventions that are accurately implemented to incur benefit. To guarantee this happens requires measuring and monitoring fidelity of implementation. Checklists for assessing fidelity listing critical steps accompany many packaged interventions. When unavailable, one can be developed based on procedural steps of the intervention. An observer then checks each step employed by the interventionist, which can be used to yield percentage fidelity for the observed session. This can be done in vivo or via video tape (pending parent consent). Chap. 6, Just-in-Time Training, focuses on promoting fidelity and reducing forgetting and offers one way to mitigate these problems and promote successful implementation.

A school mental health (SMH) professional familiar with the intervention is ideally suited to assess fidelity of others, particularly in the early phases of implementation. However, integrity should be assessed even for seasoned SMH professionals, as drift from the original intervention is common. Once interventionists have reached a high percentage integrity, periodic integrity observations are sufficient. In the absence of available SMH professionals to assess integrity on an ongoing basis, a second-best option is self-assessment. Because self-assessment is highly subject to bias (Kastorff et al., 2023), interventionists must be forthright about their own shortcomings, challenges, and potential biases during intervention implementation and supports should to be in place to assist teachers to develop needed skills (e.g., Kilic, 2016; Rispoli et al., 2017).

Although educators ideally will achieve 100% fidelity, this can be challenging. Lower fidelity (e.g., 90%) can be acceptable, provided critical components of an intervention are not omitted or incorrectly implemented. For instance, explanation of a target social skill is likely critical, while falling slightly short of praise frequency may be less consequential. When fidelity does not reach 100%, educators should identify those specific intervention steps or components they omitted or incorrectly implemented along with the reason for the lapse in fidelity, which will direct them to strategies for improvement. For example, if an interventionist is unsuccessful at teaching students how to identify their maladaptive thoughts during cognitive behavioral therapy, further training is needed. In contrast, a teacher who forgets to pre-prompt a student to engage in a particular social skill because they are busy supporting other students may just need a timer to remind them when it is time to prompt.

1.11   Assessing Intervention Impacts on Student SEBMH Functioning

Tiered systems of support are optimally effective when students seamlessly move from tier to tier or from one intervention to another within tiers. To meet this aim, the expected impact of the intervention on student concerns must be periodically assessed. Three dimensions of assessment that teams will determine include *what*, *how*, and *when* to assess. To identify *what* to assess, teams should determine student behavioral concerns that they hope to alter. It should be noted that intervention selection should be matched to student behavior need; hence, the concern the intervention is expected to impact should be one and the same as the student's challenge. However, a single intervention (e.g., cognitive behavioral intervention for depression) may have a collateral impact on related student concerns (e.g., poor academic performance, asocial behavior). In this case, it is judicious to also collect data on ancillary behaviors to ascertain the need for supplemental interventions.

When determining *how* to collect data, feasibility is a top consideration. Data that are difficult to collect, such as frequency of very high-rate behavior, is likely to be inaccurate or disregarded altogether. Many methods, such as time sampling (i.e., recording the presence or absence of behavior at predetermined timepoints), produce accurate data and render data collection practical. Further, teacher rating systems (e.g., Direct Behavior Rating; von der Embse et al., 2015), are simple and have advanced such that they are increasingly accurate and reliable measures of behavior. Although screening data might be used to determine students who need Tier 2 or Tier 3 interventions, they may not be sufficiently sensitive to pick up emotional and behavioral changes or variability in response to an intervention and additional data are recommended. For internalizing behaviors (e.g., depression, anxiety) that are not readily subject to observation, data may be collected in the form of self-report and/or through commonly implemented screening measures, which include emphases on externalizing and internalizing behaviors, as well as social functioning (see Chap. 5, this volume). This can be accompanied by any observable symptoms of behavior, such as school attendance, interactions with peers, or the frequency of requests to visit the nurse. Externalizing behaviors generally can be easily observed and recorded, such as the frequency of aggression or inappropriate peer interactions.

The final consideration is *when* to assess intervention impact. Unquestionably, baseline data should always be collected for comparison purposes. Frequent data collection (e.g., daily) allows school teams to review progress, assessing whether behavior is moving in the desired direction and intervention should be maintained. However, other factors dictate when it is most important to assess intervention effects. The duration of an intervention is one consideration. For instance, if a depression intervention spans 10 weeks, responsiveness should be assessed after students have completed the full intervention. Another consideration pertains to problem behavior history, including intensity and duration. Problem behaviors that are intransigent will be slower to respond to intervention.

1.12 Quality Assessment and Improvement Strategies

Ideas related to monitoring and improving the quality of SMH programming have been presented throughout this chapter. In our view, at the school level, perhaps the most important quality indicator is the functioning of the SEBMH lead team. Several questions should be considered to assure optimal functioning. As before, is this team inclusive of the right people, including SMH staff (school AND community-employed), educators, school administrators, allied health staff (e.g., nursing, occupational therapy), and family members and older students? Does this team meet at least twice per month? Do meetings start and end on time? Are there clear agendas, actions identified, and follow-up to these actions? Is a formal program to guide team functioning being used such as TIPS (Chaparro et al., 2022)? Is the team actively monitoring all programming across tiers, including monitoring the fidelity of, and impacts of interventions on students? Are practices being implemented indeed evidence-based? When practices do not appear to be working, are they actively adjusted, or in some cases de-implemented? Are all staff in the building knowledgeable of this team and interacting with it to provide information and observations and to ask questions?

Given this SEBMH team is well functioning (in our view, a critical lynchpin for effectiveness and scaling of SMH; Chaparro et al., 2022; Splett et al., 2017, 2024), it will be positioned to implement formal strategies for quality assessment and improvement (QAI). These include using formal measures, such as the Tiered Fidelity Inventory (TFI; https://www.pbis.org/resource/tfi); the Interconnected Systems Framework Implementation Inventory (ISFII, Splett et al., 2020), reflecting best practices in education-mental health systems integration; or the School Health and Performance Evaluation (SHAPE) system, a comprehensive QAI tool developed by the National Center on School Mental Health (NCSMH, see www.schoolmentalhealth.org). These tools are commonly completed at the beginning and end of each academic year by the SEBMH team as a group. Areas of strength and areas of weakness are identified, with quality improvement plans developed after beginning year assessment to include three to five areas for improvement, and one to two areas of strength to celebrate. At least monthly, this team should check in on progress of quality improvement targets, making adjustments in plans as indicated, with an end-of-year review of progress, which will set up repetition of this cycle building on lessons learned. Alternatively, depending on the resources of the school and functioning of the SEBMH team, these assessments can be completed annually.

As mentioned, foundational at the district level is a strong District-Community Leadership Team (DCLT) that should be monitoring what is happening in, and providing support to school buildings. As above, this team should be inclusive of the right leaders and constituents, actively monitoring and supporting best practices in school buildings, promoting sharing of lessons learned and mutual support across buildings, including identifying and sharing experiences of Model Demonstration Projects (MDPs), as well as assuring that resources at state and other levels (e.g., from federal initiatives; state, regional and national technical assistance center) are reaching and supporting the work occurring in school buildings in meaningful ways (see Eber et al., 2020).

1.13 Building Effective Vertical and Horizontal Interdisciplinary Collaboration

State to district to school building relationships and in turn, tracking progress at these levels and getting information out on best practices, and challenges and ways to overcome them (vertical collaboration) are critical to success but are often the focus on inadequate attention. Relatedly, at each of these levels, there should be strong emphases on interdisciplinary collaboration, including collaboration with families and students and other constituents (horizontal collaboration). Promoting vertical and horizontal collaboration is covered more extensively in Chap. 3 (this volume). Interested readers are also referred to a review by Weist et al. 2022b on vertical collaboration, and to Weist et al. 2012 on horizontal collaboration.

1.14 Workforce Challenges, Task Shifting, and Other Promising Strategies

Perhaps the greatest barrier to scaling effective SMH is a large and growing workforce shortage of mental health professionals. This shortage is not distributed evenly in the United States, and some geographic regions have little or no access to mental health professionals. For instance, data from the Health Resources and Services Administration (HRSA, n.d.) show that more than half of the US population, an estimated 169 million people, live in a "Mental Health Workforce Shortage Area," or an area where the population-to-provider ratio exceeds 30,000 to 1. This shortage is particularly acute in the SMH workforce, where, on average, the United States has less than half of the recommended SMH workforce supply needed to meet the demand (Sohn, 2024). Despite significant investments from the US government (e.g., the Department of Education's School-Based Mental Health Services Grant programs) designed to increase the supply of the mental health workforce, it is unlikely that such programming will satisfy the increasing demand for services, and data from HRSA's workforce projection dashboard predict increasing shortages (HRSA, n.d.). Clearly, if we are to scale effective SMH, we must scale services beyond those provided directly by traditional school behavioral health professionals. This reality reifies the importance of universal prevention and promotion efforts in the contexts of MTSS, and it also highlights the importance of novel approaches to scaling effective school behavioral health services, such as task shifting and technology-delivered interventions.

Task shifting, or the rational redistribution of tasks from professionals to helpers with less formal training or fewer credentials, is one approach to reducing the supply and demand gap in the school behavioral health workforce. Increasingly, in both domestic and global settings, mental health systems are recruiting nonexpert practitioners to broaden the reach and accessibility of mental and behavioral health services (Asnaani, 2023). An example of task shifting in the workforce is the Ballmer Institute at the University of Oregon's creation of Behavioral Health Specialists—a new bachelor's level mental health profession. This profession includes formal education through a Child Behavioral Health major at the University of Oregon, and graduates are ready to enter the school behavioral health/SMH workforce with no additional formal training. However, task-shifting efforts extend beyond the workforce and into communities, including efforts to train and equip clergy, community leaders, mentors, teachers, and peers. Collectively, efforts in task shifting are designed to increase the total volume of individuals with competencies in promoting mental health across sectors.

Schools are an ideal location to expand task-shifting efforts within the context of MTSS. First, because MTSS rely on team-based service provision, there are more professionals to oversee the supervision of shifted services. Second, schools are historically, and continue to be, hubs for community helpers, mentors, and other lay helpers or volunteers—a resource that might be leveraged to expand access to supportive services. Finally, within the context of MTSS, leveraging community or lay helpers may be one way to increase the supply of supplemental Tier 2 services. For example, Hart et al. (2021) describe a model of embedding community mentors in the context of MTSS systems, such that mentors provide supervised social, emotional, behavioral, and academic services for students with elevated needs at an appropriate level. There is emerging evidence that such task-shifting efforts are capable of promoting behavioral health outcomes, including reducing conduct problems and mental health issues, and improving grades, even among students with high levels of impairment (McQuillin & McDaniel, 2021; McQuillin et al., 2019). In summary, efforts to scale effective school mental health may need to think outside of the traditional professional helpers who provide mental health services.

1.15   Conclusion

In this chapter, we reviewed critical themes for scaling of effective SMH programs, beginning with a strong connection to schools' MTSS, and assuring the effective functioning of teams at school building, district, and state levels. Ideally, these inter-disciplinary teams are functioning effectively at each level, and actively involved in vertical collaboration across levels and horizontal collaboration within them. At the school building level, it is of foundational importance to strengthen one team focused on student social, emotional, behavioral, and mental health (SEBMH) functioning to coordinate programming within and across tiers. In turn, this team orchestrates fundamental practices including assuring broad input into school programming from diverse staff and constituents (and students and families), and leads effective core MTSS practices including data-based decision-making; installing, refining, and coaching evidence-based practices; and aligning programming across tiers, assuring equity, progress and outcome monitoring, and continuous quality improvement. At each of these levels, there is also much promise to developing model demonstration projects (MDPs), sites where best practices (as described in this chapter) are being implemented and improved, and there are methods to publicize and share experiences of these MDPs to promote collaboration, mutual support, and scaling. The remaining chapters in this book augment and amplify key themes presented in this introductory chapter.

References

Asnaani, A. (2023). What role can (and should) clinical science play in promoting mental health care equity? *American Psychologist, 78*(9), 1041–1054. https://doi.org/10.1037/amp0001217

Bal, A., Betters-Bubon, J., & Fish, R. E. (2019). A multilevel analysis of statewide disproportionality in exclusionary discipline and the identification of emotional disturbance. *Education and Urban Society, 51*(2), 247–268.

Barrett, S., Eber, L., & Weist, M. D. (2013). *Advancing education effectiveness: An interconnected systems framework for Positive Behavioral Interventions and Supports (PBIS) and school mental health.* Center for Positive Behavioral Interventions and Supports (funded by the Office of Special Education Programs, U.S. Department of Education). Eugene, Oregon, University of Oregon Press.

Benson, T. A., & Fiarman, S. E. (2020). *Unconscious bias in schools: A developmental approach to exploring race and racism.* Harvard Education Press.

Chaparro, E. A., Horner, R., Algozzine, B., Daily, J., & Nese, R. N. T. (2022). *How school teams use data to make effective decisions: Team-Initiated Problem Solving (TIPS).* University of Oregon. https://www.pbis.org

Daly, B. P., Burke, R., Hare, I., Mills, C., Owens, C., Moore, E., & Weist, M. D. (2006). Enhancing *no child left behind* – School mental health connections. *Journal of School Health, 76,* 446–451.

Eber, L., Barrett, S., Perales, K., Jeffrey-Pearsall, J., Pohlman, K., Putnam, R., Splett, J., & Weist, M. D. (2020). *Advancing education effectiveness: Interconnecting school mental health and school-wide PBIS, Volume 2: An implementation guide.* Center for Positive Behavioral Interventions and Supports (funded by the Office of Special Education Programs, U.S. Department of Education). Eugene, Oregon: University of Oregon Press.

George, M. R., Taylor, L. K., Schmidt, S., & Weist, M. D. (2013). A review of school mental health programs in SAMHSA's National Registry of Evidence-Based Programs and Practices. *Psychiatric Services, 64*(5), 483–486.

Hart, M., Flitner, A., Kornbluh, M., Thompson, D., Davis, A., Lanza-Gregory, J., McQuillin, S., Gonzalez, J., & Strait, G. (2021). Combining MTSS and community-based mentoring programs. *School Psychology Review.* https://doi.org/10.1080/2372966X.2021.1922937

Hawken, L. S., Bundock, K., Kladis, K., O'Keeffe, B., & Barrett, C. A. (2014). Systematic Review of the Check-in, Check-out Intervention for Students At Risk for Emotional and Behavioral Disorders. *Education and Treatment of Children 37*(4), 635–658. https://doi.org/10.1353/etc.2014.0030

Health Resources and Services Administration. (n.d.). *Projecting the supply and demand of health professionals: 2018–2030.* Retrieved from https://bhw.hrsa.gov/data-research/projecting-health-workforce-supply-demand

Kastorff, T., Sailer, M., Vejvoda, J., Schultz-Pernice, F., Hartmann, V., Hertl, A., et al. (2023). Context-specificity to reduce bias in self-assessments: Comparing teachers' scenario-based self-assessment and objective assessment of technological knowledge. *Journal of Research on Technology in Education, 55*(6), 917–930.

Kern, L., George, M., & Weist, M. D. (2016). *Step by step support for students with emotional and behavioral problems: Prevention and intervention strategies.* Brookes Publishing.

Kern, L., Gaier, K., Kelly, S., Nielsen, C. M., Commisso, C. E., & Wehby, J. H. (2020). An evaluation of adaptations made to Tier 2 social skill training programs. *Journal of Applied School Psychology, 36*(2), 155–172.

Kilic, D. (2016). An examination of using self-, peer-, and teacher-assessment in higher education: A case study in teacher education. *Higher Education Studies, 6*(1), 136–144.

Kittelman, A., Mercer, S. H., McIntosh, K., Morris, K. R., & Hatton, H. L. (2023). Validation of a measure of district systems implementation of Positive Behavioral Interventions and Supports. *Remedial and Special Education, 44*(4), 259–271. https://doi.org/10.1177/07419325221114472

Lyon, A. R., Bruns, E.J., Ludwig, K. et al. (2015). The Brief Intervention for School Clinicians (BRISC): A Mixed-Methods Evaluation of Feasibility, Acceptability, and Contextual Appropriateness. *School Mental Health 7*, 273–286. https://doi.org/10.1007/s12310-015-9153-0

Majeika, C. E., Van Camp, A. M., Wehby, J. H., Kern, L., Commisso, C. E., & Gaier, K. (2020). An evaluation of adaptations made to Check-In Check-Out. *Journal of Positive Behavior Interventions, 22*, 25–37.

McIntosh, K., Ellwood, K., McCall, L., & Girvan, E. J. (2018). Using Discipline Data to Enhance Equity in School Discipline. *Intervention in School and Clinic, 53*(3), 146–152. https://doi.org/10.1177/1053451217702130

McNeill, K. F., Friedman, B. D., & Chavez, C. (2016). Keep them so you can teach them: Alternatives to exclusionary discipline. *International Public Health Journal, 8*(2), 169–181.

McQuillin, S. D., & McDaniel, H. L. (2021). Pilot randomized trial of brief school-based mentoring for middle school students with elevated disruptive behavior. *Annals of the New York Academy of Sciences, 1483*(1), 127–141. https://doi.org/10.1111/nyas.14334

McQuillin, S. D., Lyons, M. D., Becker, K. D., Hart, M. J., & Cohen, K. (2019). Strengthening and expanding child services in low resource communities: The role of task-shifting and just-in-time training. *American journal of community psychology, 63*(3–4), 355–365. https://doi.org/10.1002/ajcp.12314

Oakes, W. P., Lane, K. L., Cantwell, E. D., & Royer, D. J. (2017). Systematic screening for behavior in K-12 settings as regular school practice: Practical considerations and recommendations. *Journal of Applied School Psychology, 33*, 369–393. https://doi.org/10.1080/15377903.2017.1345813

Rispoli, M., Zaini, S., Mason, R., Brodhead, M., Burke, M. D., & Gregori, E. (2017). A systematic review of teacher self-monitoring on implementation of behavioral practices. *Teaching and Teacher Education, 63*, 58–72.

Sohn, E. (2024, January 1). There's a strong push for more school psychologists. *Monitor on Psychology, 55*(1) https://www.apa.org/monitor/2024/01/trends-more-school-psychologists-needed

Splett, J. W., Perales, K., Halliday-Boykins, C. A., Gilchrest, C., Gibson, N., & Weist, M. D. (2017). Best practices for teaming and collaboration in the Interconnected Systems Framework. *Journal of Applied School Psychology, 33*(4), 347–368.

Splett, J. W., Trainor, K., Raborn, A., Halliday-Boykins, C., Garzona, M., Dongo, M., & Weist, M. D. (2018). Comparison of universal mental health screening and traditional school identification methods for multi-tiered intervention planning. *Behavioral Disorders, 43*(3), 344–356.

Splett, J. W., Perales, K., Al-Khatib, A., Raborn, A., & Weist, M. D. (2020). Preliminary development and validation of the Interconnected Systems Framework Implementation Inventory (ISF-II). *School Psychology, 35*(4), 255–266.

Splett, J. W., Perales, K., Pohlman, K., Alquiza, K., Collins, D., Gomez, N., Houston-Dial, R., Meyer, B., & Weist, M. D. (2024). *Enhancing team functioning in schools' multi-tiered systems of support*. Center for Positive Behavioral Interventions and Supports (funded by the Office of Special Education Programs, U.S. Department of Education). Eugene, Oregon: University of Oregon Press. Retrieved from http://www.pbis.org

Tefera, A. A., & Fischman, G. E. (2020). How and why context matters in the study of racial disproportionality in special education: Toward a critical disability education policy approach. *Equity & Excellence in Education, 53*(4), 433–448.

von der Embse, N., Scott, E. C., & Kilgus, S. P. (2015). The sensitivity to change and concurrent validity of direct behavior rating single item scales for anxiety. *School Psychology Quarterly, 30*, 244–259. https://doi.org/10.1037/spq0000083

von der Embse, N. P., Kilgus, S. P., Eklund, K., Ake, E., & Levi-Neilsen, S. (2018). Training teachers to facilitate early identification of mental and behavioral health risks. *School Psychology Review, 47*(4), 372–384.

Weist, M. D., Rubin, M., Moore, E., Adelsheim, S., & Wrobel, G. (2007). Mental health screening in schools. *Journal of School Health, 77*, 53–58.

Weist, M. D., Paternite, C. E., Wheatley-Rowe, D., & Gall, G. (2009). From thought to action in school mental health promotion. *International Journal of Mental Health Promotion, 11*(3), 32–41.

Weist, M. D., Mellin, E. A., Chambers, K., Lever, N. A., Haber, D., & Blaber, C. (2012). Challenges to collaboration in school mental health and strategies for overcoming them. *Journal of School Health, 82*(2), 97–105.

Weist, M. D., Garbacz, A., Lane, K. E., & Kincaid, D. (2017). *Aligning and integrating family engagement in Positive Behavioral Interventions and Supports (PBIS): Concepts and strategies for families and schools in key contexts*. Center for Positive Behavioral Interventions and Supports (funded by the Office of Special Education Programs, U.S. Department of Education). Eugene, Oregon: University of Oregon Press.

Weist, M. D., Eber, L., Horner, R., Splett, J., Putnam, R., Barrett, S., Perales, K., Fairchild, A. J., & Hoover, S. (2018). Improving multi-tiered systems of support for students with "internalizing" emotional/behavioral problems. *Journal of Positive Behavior Interventions, 20*(3), 172–184.

Weist, M. D., Splett, J. W., Halliday, C., Gage, N. A., Seaman, M., Perkins, K., Perales, K., Miller, E., Collins, D., & Distefano, C. (2022a). A randomized controlled trial on the Interconnected Systems Framework for School Mental Health and PBIS: Focus on proximal variables and school discipline. *Journal of School Psychology, 94*, 49–65.

Weist, M. D., Figas, K., Stern, K., Terry, J., Scherder, E., Collins, D., Davis, T., & Stevens, R. (2022b). Advancing school behavioral health at multiple levels of scale. *Pediatric Clinics of North America, 69*(4), 725–737.

Chapter 2
Tiered Mental Health Support: Meeting the Needs of All Students

Lee Kern and Leigh Kuenne Rusnak

2.1 Introduction to Tiered Support

The concept of multitiered systems of support (MTSS) traces back to the field of public health. Within this domain, the focus was prevention and treatment of disease and other health concerns. The public health system relied on three tiers, a configuration that has been maintained with expanded applications. Tier 1 focuses on primary prevention, averting health problems by addressing their root causes through strategies that increase resistance to disease and injury (e.g., reducing second-hand smoke, vaccinating, requiring seat belt use). Tier 2, or secondary prevention, reduces the effects of disease or injury in early stages (e.g., supporting tobacco cessation, antibiotic treatment). The goal of Tier 3, known as tertiary prevention, is to reduce the effects of an illness or injury and prevent its recurrence. Examples include coronary artery bypass surgery, burn treatment, and neurosurgery. This model was vastly successful, particularly for reducing mortality and increasing life expectancy (e.g., Grove & Hetzel, 1968) and proved to be efficient and cost-effective.

About two decades ago, the model was introduced in school settings. At that time, schools were well positioned to replace the "wait to fail" approach whereby students received support only after their learning, behavioral, or emotional health became significantly discrepant from their peers. Predictably, waiting until students failed left them without support to remedy more minor problems, which usually escalated in severity. Tiered support offered an alternative that hinged on prevention, avoided delays to receiving intervention, and was cost-effective in a system with finite resources.

MTSS was initially applied in educational settings in the form of Response to Intervention (RtI), which focused on academics (Fletcher & Vaughn, 2009).

L. Kern (✉) · L. K. Rusnak
Lehigh University, Bethlehem, PA, USA
e-mail: lek6@lehigh.edu; lnr293@lehigh.edu

The goal was to address the presumed over-identification of students as learning disabled. In addition, RtI turned attention to the notion that inadequate general education instruction was responsible for excessive numbers of students receiving labels of learning disability. The intention of RtI was to create a continuum of instructional supports to prevent academic failure that would replace the foregoing two-option model of general and special education.

Subsequent to the introduction of RtI, tiered models were developed in the area of emotional and behavioral health, the most prevalent and well researched being School-Wide Positive Behavior Support (SWPBS). Numerous studies, including rigorous randomized controlled trials, have substantiated the effectiveness of SWPBIS, not only for reducing behavioral problems, but also for its economy of resources (e.g., Lee & Gage, 2020). Although SWPBIS initially focused on preventing or decreasing incidents of externalizing or acting out problems (e.g., aggression, disruption, disrespectful comments), recent iterations fully embed interventions for internalizing and mental health concerns (depression, anxiety; Weist et al., 2018), primarily through Communities of Practice and the Interconnected Systems Framework (see Chap. 3, this volume). Further, because internalizing problems are inherently difficult to identify, universal screening (see Chap. 5, this volume) is used to complement traditional detection processes (e.g., office disciplinary referrals) for identifying students who would benefit from support at each tier.

Designing and sustaining a tiered mental health system is not an easy endeavor. It requires organizational structure as well as collective and collaborative engagement of all adults in the school setting as well as community constituents. A strong sense of *psychological ownership* (Dawkins et al., 2017), in which individuals identify with their school and feel a sense of belonging and effectiveness, is elemental to a well-functioning tiered system. In this chapter, we describe tiered support as contextualized through a mental health lens. In addition, we emphasize the merit of this approach for scaling school mental health.

2.2 The Tiered Framework

The expectation of tiered supports, as an efficient system of prevention, is that diminishing numbers of students will require support as tiers increase in intensity, as depicted in Fig. 2.1. As noted above, and consistent with the public health conceptualization, all students in a school receive Tier 1, or universal intervention. Tier 2 is used with students who are not sufficiently responsive to Tier 1. Tier 3 is reserved for yet a smaller percentage of students with the most intensive support needs. Initial estimates, derived from the public health framework, placed approximately 10–15% of students at a given school at Tier 2 and 3–5% at Tier 3. Recent epidemiological data, coupled with school-wide screening results, indicate these data greatly underestimate the social, emotional, and behavioral health challenges experienced by school-age students, particularly subsequent to COVID (Weist et al., 2023). For instance, in the year following the COVID lockdown, approximately

Fig. 2.1 Illustration of tiered support

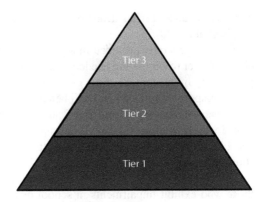

25% of youth experienced depression at a clinically significant level (National Academies of Sciences, Engineering, and Medicine, 2023). This figure is five times prior estimates of students needing Tier 3 intervention.

Another consideration is the additional variables that play a role in student responsiveness to intervention, which in turn alters the number of students requiring Tier 2 and 3 interventions. These include integrity of intervention implementation (i.e., the extent interventions were implemented as designed), the extensiveness of screening for identification of students who would benefit from support, and contextual variables surrounding the school (e.g., poverty, community safety, exposure to adverse childhood experiences), to note just a few. These increased percentages of student challenges have resource implications, and policy considerations should follow to ensure resource adequacy. Therefore, we advise school staff to consider both internal/local and external contextual factors and plan accordingly.

2.2.1   Overview of Each Tier

Tier 1 support is intended for *all* students. Consistent with a preventive purpose, intervention at this tier targets the broad skills that students need for productive social, emotional, and behavioral functioning and well-being. It is important to note that skills at Tier 1 are taught and reinforced, as there is no assumption that students come to school already possessing such skills. Instruction that emphasizes emotional and behavioral health includes mental health education lessons and social-emotional learning. An important agenda of mental health education is to reduce the lingering stigma regarding mental health concerns. Further, emotional and behavioral health targets teachers and staff as well, for whom stress and other mental health-related variables interfere with effective teaching, hinder productive teacher-student relationships, and lead to teacher attrition (Agyapong et al., 2022). Finally, improving school climate also is a target of Tier 1 intervention. Improvements in this area are associated with a number of advantageous student outcomes, including better attendance, higher academic achievement, and greater rates of graduation (Daily et al., 2020).

Tier 2 is generally provided in a group context for the purpose of resource efficiency. Fewer resources are needed when students can be clustered for intervention, particularly in the context of the growing percentage of students who are not sufficiently responsive to Tier 1 and will benefit from additional support. Although some students may require ongoing Tier 2 support, many need only short-term interventions focused on topical issues, such as grief following the death of a family member. Efficiency also is exercised when students with similar needs are grouped for short-term support.

Students experiencing significant mental and behavioral health concerns, and those who exhibit impairments in school or personal functioning, required Tier 3 intervention. Tier 3 mental health support is generally provided by school mental health professionals who are either employed by the school or collaborating community providers (see Chap. 1, this volume). Support at this level is individualized, often relying on a functional behavioral assessment to ascertain environmental changes that can be made to support the individual, coupled with mental health assessments to identify underlying challenges. The typically complex concerns of students requiring intensive supports almost always dictate the need for a multicomponent support plan. Effective supports may often go beyond the school setting and incorporate family therapy, interventions to enhance the student's quality of life, and (for adolescents) planning for the future.

2.3   Examples of Interventions at Each Tier

The literature is now replete with research supporting the effectiveness of a variety of interventions at each tier for reducing student emotional and behavioral challenges. As noted above, many interventions have targeted externalizing, or acting out behaviors. An example of the most common Tier 1 intervention is issuing rewards for students who are following school-wide expectations. Although interventions of this nature are important, they fail to fully address the many mental health problems common among children and adolescents. Consequently, as tiered systems have evolved, they have increasingly integrated mental health interventions and supports. In the following sections, we describe supports focused on healthy emotional development. In addition, we describe the ways in which common behavioral interventions have expanded to address student mental health needs.

2.3.1 Tier 1 Intervention

As noted above, Tier 1 school-based mental health interventions and services prioritize the promotion of emotional and behavioral health and the prevention of mental health challenges for all students. Designed to provide universal support, interventions aim to explicitly teach social, emotional, and behavioral skills that foster overall well-being and lead to academic progress. A collateral goal is successful transition to adulthood. When effective, Tier 1 services embody a multifaceted approach that fosters a culturally and linguistically inclusive school climate, allowing the majority of students to be successful academically, socially, and behaviorally.

The School Mental Health Quality Guide, developed by the University of Maryland School of Medicine (National Center for School Mental Health, 2023), recommended a number of Tier 1 services and supports to promote schools mental health. Included among those recommendations are assessing and improving school climate, evaluating and improving teacher and school staff well-being, establishing school-wide expectations and associated systems of positive reinforcement that reduce exclusionary approaches, increasing mental health literacy among both students and staff, and increasing social and emotional learning skills. They further recommend relying on Tier 1 services and supports that are evidence-based, equitable, and address the needs of students and their families. Below we briefly describe these practices.

School climate is a multifaceted concept comprising diverse aspects of the educational experience. Building a positive school climate includes focus on strong academics, productive relationships among all constituents, and a feeling of safety. Programs that support student voice and choice such as mentoring, peer-conflict resolution, and extra- and co-curricular clubs and activities (e.g., student council) contribute to students feeling seen and heard in the school environment. School climate data, most commonly measured by student and staff surveys, inform the nature of interventions needed for all constituents, students, staff, and families to feel positive about the quality and character of school life (National School Climate Center, 2021).

Linked to school climate is teacher and staff well-being. Emotionally healthy adults are prepared to support students' emotional regulation, engage students in learning, and recognize signs of student distress (Yanek et al., 2022). Conversely, research has shown that when teachers experience mental health concerns, it impacts the overall quality of instruction provided to students and, hence, student outcomes (McLean et al., 2017). Similar to youth-targeted interventions, meta-analyses (e.g., von der Embse et al., 2019) suggest diverse approaches are effective at reducing staff stress and burnout and improving mental health. The most common include cognitive behavioral therapy, relaxation, meditation, mindfulness approaches (e.g., yoga), and interventions that focus on improving student behavior.

Establishing clear expectations and rewarding students for following those expectations is a fundamental Tier 1 strategy that forms the foundation for positive discipline among all school community members. Knowing what is expected and the consequences of meeting those expectations creates a sense of structure and predictability for students as well as a managed and productive environment for learning. Strong relationships arise from the positive interactions between students and staff as students are rewarded for appropriate behavior and, when extended to the classroom, allow a place of comfort, cooperation, and open communication (Minahan, 2019). When students present with challenging behaviors that violate school-wide expectations, a consistent and constructive approach designed to teach and encourage appropriate behavior (as opposed to using punitive and exclusionary methods) provides support for overall student mental health (Reinert et al., 2022).

Mental health literacy is an essential Tier 1 support that is most successful when it targets all school constituents, including students, teachers, staff, and parents. Simply defined, mental health literacy aims to strengthen knowledge and beliefs about mental health challenges to increase recognition, prevention, and management. Improved literacy leads to a better educated school community that can prevent mental health concerns from going unnoticed and reduce associated stigma (for more details, see School Mental Health Quality Guide, 2023). Several mental health literacy programs are available free of charge, including Classroom Wise (https://www.classroomwise.org) and Headstrong (Perry et al., 2014; https://www.blackdoginstitute.org.au/education-services/schools/school-resources/headstrong/).

Finally, because social-emotional learning (SEL) is integral to child development, Tier 1 instruction in this area is intended to enhance student self-awareness, self-management, social awareness, relationship skills, and responsible decision-making (Collaborative for Academic, Social, and Emotional Learning [CASEL], 2022). These skills, in turn, promote academic and social success. Several evidence-based SEL programs are readily available for use in school contexts (e.g., PeaceWorks, Responsive Classroom, Second Step®). Further, these programs should be combined with school-wide practices (e.g., staff modeling coping strategies) to promote SEL in authentic situations (CASEL, 2022).

As noted in Chap. 1 (this volume), a social, emotional, behavioral, and mental health (SEBMH) lead team, consisting of administrators, teachers, parents, and students, oversees the creation and execution of a cohesive system of Tier 1 supports. Data allow the SEBMH team to generate a hierarchy of school needs to prioritize intervention selection and implementation. Relevant data include attendance information, climate surveys, disciplinary referrals, and screening outcomes. These data allow for a tailored approach to Tier 1. A well-functioning array of Tier 1 supports customized to each school community reaches the majority of students in a school. In turn, this creates a foundation for identifying students experiencing more serious mental health challenges.

2.3.2 Tier 2 Intervention

The three most common Tier 2 interventions are Check In-Check-Out (CICO), social skills groups, and self-management (Bruhn et al., 2014; Cho Blair et al., 2021). Each benefits from substantial research support. They are relatively easy to implement in that they can be seamlessly blended into the ongoing daily school routine, in the case of CICO and self-management, or can be conducted in a group format, as in social skills groups, thereby simultaneously addressing the needs of multiple students.

In brief, CICO (Hawken et al., 2020) is a structured intervention in which students check in with a mentor at the start of the school day to receive a daily progress report (DPR) and establish goals for the day ahead. Goals generally align with the school-wide expectations but can be adapted to address individual student needs, including internalizing problems, as we illustrate below. The student then carries the DPR throughout the day, receiving points at pre-designated times for following the listed expectations. At the end of the school day, the student again meets with their mentor to review their earned points, receiving praise and perhaps a reward for meeting a previously established daily goal (e.g., earning 80% of points). If the goal was not met, the mentor offers feedback and discussion about behaviors needed to meet their goal in the future. To establish a home-school connection, the student then takes the DPR home, with the expectation that a parent/guardian will provide praise, feedback, and encouragement. The student returns the DPR the following morning, signed by the parent/guardian, and the cycle resumes.

As noted above, in addition to reducing acting out behaviors, research also demonstrates that CICO is effective for students with internalizing problems (Kladis et al., 2023). For example, Mitchell et al. (2021) made simple adaptations to goals on the daily progress report to align with the needs of participants with anxiety, depression, and somatization, such as participating in class activities and discussion, persisting with difficult tasks, and seeking assistance when needed. The adapted CICO resulted in increases in academic engaged time and reductions in teacher-rated internalizing problems. Hunter et al. (2014) made an adaptation to the morning check-in meeting to address internalizing problems. With support from their mentors, students identified their maladaptive and negative patterns of thinking and generated ways to replace the negative thoughts with those that were positive and productive and/or invoke problem-solving strategies. The intervention was followed by improved behavior, as measured by DPR data, and for the majority of participants, reductions in internalizing behaviors as measured by screener scores.

Another common Tier 2 intervention is social skills groups. Numerous social skills curricula are commercially available. Recent research has illustrated ways to both enhance their effectiveness and render them more efficient. One strategy is to group students with similar concerns (e.g., anxiety) and provide targeted intervention. A second approach is to identify specific student skill challenges and deliver intervention that targets those challenges. For instance, students who have difficulty with turn taking can be grouped for skill instruction in this area. Third, because group-based social skills are typically provided outside of the typical settings in which social problems occur (e.g., classroom, playground), practitioners in natural settings (e.g., teachers, parents, sometimes peers) should prompt and reinforce use of the skills learned. This is particularly important for single session interventions (see Chap. 7, this volume).

Self-management, a third prevalent Tier 2 strategy, involves teaching students to observe occurrences of their own behavior or thoughts, compare their behavior to a pre-established goal or standard, and self-reinforce when the goal is achieved. Self-management interventions largely address externalizing problem behaviors, with on-task behavior the most common intervention target (Briesch & Briesch, 2016). However, a few studies have demonstrated that it can be used effectively with a variety of internalizing problems. For instance, following direct instruction in the use of social skills, Marchant et al. (2007) taught socially withdrawn elementary-aged students to self-monitor their effective communication and appropriate peer play on the playground, with resulting improvements in both behaviors. Similarly, Kauer et al. (2012) taught adolescents to self-monitor their mood, stress, and use of coping strategies, resulting in significant decreases in depressive symptoms. Self-management also can be embedded within other Tier 2 interventions, such as relaxation training, to assist children to self-monitor both their internal states and their subsequent use of strategies, when needed (Zakszeski et al., 2023).

Additional Tier 2 interventions continue to emerge. For instance, single session interventions (see Chap. 7, this volume) are rapidly gathering research evidence. Additional interventions identified in a recent meta-analysis (Cho Blair et al., 2021) include Breaks are Better, a modification of CICO, aimed at students who engage in behavior to escape tasks, assignments, or activities, and Class Pass in which students are permitted to appropriately request a limited number of breaks. Further, variations of CICO, such as using peers for intervention implementation, have growing prevalence in both research and practice.

2.3.3   Tier 3 Intervention

Tier 3 intervention is individualized and generally relies on information derived from a functional behavioral assessment (FBA). A comprehensive FBA identifies not only environmental events associated with problem behavior, but also underlying issues that contribute to problem behavior (e.g., post-traumatic stress disorder; Bambara & Kern, 2021). Mental health assessments, such as anxiety or depression inventories, should complement an FBA to identify related programs and supports that a student may need. A multicomponent support plan is then developed that directly links to the FBA findings and results of the mental health assessment. The plan should contain preventive interventions, socially appropriate behaviors to replace problematic behaviors, strategies for adults to respond to problem behavior that are instructive and unlikely to reinforce the behavior, targeted mental health programs, and quality of life interventions (Bambara & Kern, 2021). Because a thorough description of the process for Tier 3 assessment and support plan development exceeds the scope of this chapter, we refer readers to other sources (e.g., Bambara & Kern, 2021).

Evidence-based interventions should be implemented when specific mental health challenges are identified. Examples include Cognitive Behavioral Therapy (CBT), Trauma-Focused CBT (Thielemann, et al., 2022), and Interpersonal Skills Training (see https://www.pbis.org/pbis/tier-2). Within the broader child and mental health field, there is significant movement toward modular EBPs (Lucassen et al., 2015). For example, the MATCH-ADTC resource, available via the PracticeWise system (https://www.practicewise.com/), provides practical guidance for implementing practice elements with the most empirical support for the highest prevalence youth mental health disorders of anxiety, depression, trauma, and conduct problems. For example, top practice elements for anxiety include cognitive coping, relaxation, and exposure. Particular caution is needed at Tier 3 as there are a range of practices used by mental health professionals that have little or no empirical support, such as psychodynamic therapies.

2.4   Aligning Programming Across Tiers

Although the previous sections described interventions specific to each tier, a critical feature of well-done MTSS (as in PBIS) is aligning programming across tiers. That is, an emphasis is on systematic connections between programs at each of the three tiers, versus separate, disconnected programming. Tier 1 represents the foundation for all programming and as mentioned, includes universal programming for all students, and infrastructure and strategies for key MTSS practices (e.g., teams; data-based decision-making; installing, evaluating, improving evidence-based practices; providing coaching support; progress monitoring). As part of Tier 1 core practices, there should be a focus on assuring connections between programming at tiers, and assuring that practices at each tier support practices in the other two. For example, if a community is experiencing a high level of trauma (e.g., natural disaster, school shooting, student suicide), the emphasis should not just be on strengthening Tier 3 intervention program to assist traumatized youth, but strengthening programming at all tiers.

In this example, Tier 1 programming could be strengthened through a focus on mental health literacy (see Kutcher et al., 2013) emphasizing the impact of trauma on students, families, and school staff. Such programming may have a number of expected benefits including reducing stigma, promoting help-seeking, and resulting in therapeutic impacts (e.g., learning about Post-Traumatic Stress Disorder [PTSD]) and trauma symptoms can be therapeutic for people experiencing these symptoms (Gee et al., 2020). This school/district could also choose to implement the program, Supporting Students Exposed to Trauma (SSET; Jaycox et al., 2009), a classroom-based program helping students navigate through the experience of trauma. A more intensive program involving small group intervention, the Cognitive Behavioral

Intervention for Trauma in Schools (CBITS, Nadeem et al., 2014), could span Tiers 2 and 3 for students experiencing more intensive trauma symptoms. Students with diagnoses of PTSD could also receive individual family therapy through Trauma-Focused CBT (Connors et al., 2021). The SEBMH lead team in the school would track implementation of each of these programs, monitoring their fidelity and impact, and use these data to connect students to appropriate programming at each tier. Importantly, such programming should not be viewed as mutually exclusive, as all students would benefit from universal MHL programming, and those with more intensive needs from the Tiers 2 and 3 programs. Some students will benefit from involvement in both SSET and CBITS and/or Trauma-Focused CBT. Given resource constraints in schools, and again using progress monitoring data, it would be incumbent on the SEBMH team to make the most effective decisions on if/when some students will receive combined programming at Tiers 2 and 3. The important point is that through using tiered logic, the SEBMH team focuses on strengthening appropriate programming at each tier, with the prediction that enhancements in Tier 1 programming will reduce Tier 2 and Tier 3 needs, and in turn, strengthening Tier 2 programming will reduce Tier 3 needs.

2.5 Tier Placement and Movement

A method for identifying students who need supports at each tier is essential for the success of a structured tiered system of supports. This involves determining what data will be collected, how they will be gathered, how they will be shared, and when they will be reviewed and revisited. Data review and decision-making is best accomplished by relying on the SEBMH lead team, assembled for the purpose of programming across tiers (see Chaps. 1 and 3, this volume). The SEBMH team should include school counselors, administrators, and representative teachers, and students in collaboration with community partners (e.g., local mental health liaisons). The team is charged with both identifying student support needs and managing student movement across tiers. During regular meetings, data-based decisions are made about student needs, tier placement, and movement between tiers. Data for placement, monitoring, and movement through the tiers is most efficient if it capitalizes on existing systems, resources, and processes.

To determine the initial tier placement, the SEBMH team collaboratively examines data to ascertain each student's current levels of need. It is best to rely on multiple sources of data to accurately and comprehensively identify student need not only initially but as students' mental health profiles change. Student grades are an excellent source of data for assessing connectedness and engagement in academics. Behavioral data, such as office referrals and classroom incidents, offer insight into a student's readiness to learn. Attendance concerns may indicate withdrawal or possible depression. The Student Information Systems (SIS) can typically be used to identify students who exhibit risk factors in academic, disciplinary, or attendance domains, allowing the SEBMH team to place students in the appropriate tier.

Additionally, teacher and school counselor observational input, and parent requests for assistance may influence student placement through qualitative feedback from students' closest relationships.

Universal screeners (see Chap. 5, this volume) also play an important role in determining the overall needs of the student population and inform schools about how to allocate resources based on the student population's areas of challenge. Importantly, screeners provide information about students who are at-risk and need additional supports, as well as the type of support needed, so that intervention can be initiated without waiting for significant symptoms to arise. In addition, they may identify students with serious mental health concerns who need Tier 3 intensive mental health supports (Center for School Mental Health, 2018).

Ongoing evaluation, in the form of progress monitoring, reveals student progress toward goals. For example, a student experiencing depression in the form of withdrawal behaviors, such as poor attendance and lack of engagement in academic work, may participate in a Tier 2 academic skills group and Tier 3 cognitive behavioral therapy. Because responsiveness is expected within a period of eight weeks, the student's goal is being present for 90% of school days across four weeks and no grades lower than a C on homework, classwork, and tests. Hence, progress is reviewed after eight weeks to determine whether the interventions are effective and should be maintained or need to be altered. As the student makes progress toward more consistent attendance and better academic performance, the SEBMH or Tier team might consider fading supports while monitoring to assure improvements continue.

Movement across tiers should be a fluid process, with teams continuously monitoring and regularly assessing student progress. As students make improvements, supports should be faded. Conversely, if students experience regression, the team should consider whether more or different supports are needed or if the student should move to a higher tier.

2.6   Establishing and Sustaining Systemic Supports

School systems have increasingly recognized the diverse needs of students and their obligation to provide multiple resources and programs to support school-based mental health. A shared belief in the need for school-based mental health is a concept espoused by the National Alliance on Mental Illness (NAMI, n.d.) and endorsed by parents, the National Education Association https://www.nea.org/ and in ref National Education Association (NEA) https://www.nea.org/, and the American Federation of Teachers (AFT, n.d.). Many schools have been successful in creating tiered systems that effectively connect struggling students with the supports they need. This, however, requires engagement from all constituents, training, and resource management to maximize effectiveness.

Building an organizational structure to establish and sustain a tiered mental health system depends on the collective and collaborative engagement of all adults in the school setting as well as community constituents. School staff need to comply with processes for administering screeners, follow procedures for referrals, supply data about students, implement intervention, and progress monitor students receiving Tier 2 and 3 supports. Administration must be diligent in supervision of the processes, ensuring that all teams have time to regularly meet and that fidelity of programs is upheld. Community partners and outside services must be reliable with their delivery of services and effectively communicate with the school staff. To create this synergistic community, all participants need to feel ownership.

Psychological ownership describes a person's attachment to their organization and its initiatives through the domains of efficacy, self-identity, and belongingness (Dawkins et al., 2017) and is essential for building a well-functioning tiered system. Efficacy of the MTSS system is dependent on constituents feeling a sense of influence over the mental health of their students. A sense of efficacy can be built by tapping into the shared belief of the need to support student mental health and highlighting the necessity of teachers and administrators to leverage their knowledge and relationships with students. Acknowledging staff who are committed to Tier 1 interventions and sharing student successes can contribute to their feelings of efficacy and increase implementation with fidelity.

Self-identity manifests when individual school staff perceive the duty to support student mental wellness as "theirs." Staff must understand their responsibility to implement the system in order to achieve the goal of healthier students. When leadership recognizes and reinforces the contributions of staff to the system, the significance of the responsibility builds feelings of pride. Systemic change requires administrators who faithfully meet with the staff, monitor implementation, and track student data, which in turn enhances staff sense of self and their role in promoting student mental health.

It is essential for each constituent to understand their individual role in the system, which also builds a feeling of belongingness. Identifying the roles and responsibilities of each person in the system calls attention to the interconnectedness of all parties and the crucial nature of each individual to the goal of student mental health. For example, highlighting the indispensable counseling services for a student helps a community partner discern their belonging to the overall system. Combined efforts must be made to build all partners' feelings of efficacy, self-identity, and belongingness to the school-based mental health structure, which results in a strong commitment to serve students.

It also is critical for constituents to fully understand the structure of the tiered mental health system, which requires documentation and training. Compiling written diagrams and manuals of processes and procedures must be done early in the development of the system. For instance, common vocabulary, workflows, descriptions of the tiers, and supports the school or district offers within each tier should be defined and readily available for reference by the staff and community partners. Internal websites and electronic documents are advantageous as they allow staff to edit and update supports that may change due to availability or need. A cadre of training materials can be built by creating thorough definitions and descriptions of the system, including the vision, goals, and expected outcomes.

A systemic approach to school-based mental health can be introduced using the typical professional development structures within a school district. The top leadership of the district sets the vision of providing a safe and supportive system for promoting mental health and wellness and imparts the importance of this initiative. A superintendent who connects the tiered support framework to the mission and vision of the entire district enables the training of details to bear significance.

2.7 Creating a Context for Tiered Mental Health Support

As we noted above, tiered support is an efficient approach for assuring that support reaches all students. Further, although much work lies ahead, its flexibility allows schools to respond to the rapidly changing demographics of the United States. This includes the unique challenges faced by particular student subgroups (e.g., LGBTQ, intersecting identities, immigrants [as described in Chap. 8, this volume]). National data (e.g., Adolescent and School Health (DASH) | CDC, n.d) clearly show that student mental health problems are on the rise, particularly among such subgroups. As schools are uniquely positioned to best deliver mental health supports, a few additional contextual features can facilitate the seamless delivery of effective intervention.

2.7.1 Blending Systems of Support

Existing systems of support within a school (e.g., academic, emotional/behavioral, community mental health) may be blended or merged, with many resultant benefits. First, such an approach considers student needs in a holistic fashion. For instance, many academic problems stem from unaddressed emotional challenges. An ideal intervention will jointly remediate both issues. Second, cooperative teaming encourages common language and structure. Third, merging support systems can increase intervention efficiency and effectiveness by reducing redundancy and identifying complementary interventions to maximize intervention effects. Finally, when the time and efforts of multiple teams are reduced, systems have a greater likelihood of sustainability.

To initiate system integration, teams evaluate both the way they review data and the interventions that each student receives. Student data should be reviewed collectively to ascertain not only the manifestation of student problems (e.g., failing grades) but also the underlying causes (e.g., depression). In addition, teams should examine the theory underlying each intervention approach offered within the various systems to identify both shared and unique components. Shared components of theoretically similar interventions can be eliminated while divergent and synergistic components are maintained.

2.7.2 Establishing Efficient School Teams

We have mentioned teams throughout this chapter and suggested, in the previous section, the benefits of combining systems of support and their respective teams. Schools often have a multitude of teams that perform various functions. Although it may be important to maintain certain teams (e.g., SEBMH lead team), others might be combined or even eliminated. As noted above, the function and purpose of teams should be identified. We recommend relying on the resource mapping process, as detailed in Chap. 4 (this volume). For example, during the resource mapping process, the purpose of each team can be assessed to identify overlap, eliminating redundancy or combining teams when collective decision-making is advantageous.

2.7.3 Wellness Centers

Wellness Centers provide a centralized space for the implementation of a variety of evidence-based practices that lead to improved mental health of students. These sites are designed to support all students in managing their mental health needs and provide a place to implement interventions for students requiring higher-tiered services (Wang et al., 2020). School-based Wellness Centers typically offer a tranquil space for students who may experience stress during their school day. Rooms may include sensory activities and provide space for meditation and emotional de-escalation. Some Wellness Centers are staffed with personnel who assist in structuring the de-escalation process or connecting students with resources, such as counseling or occupational therapy for sensory needs. The center is a hub for students in need of all tiers of support.

Wellness Centers can serve multiple capacities within a school-based mental health system (Wang et al., 2020). The Wellness Center can function in a Tier 1 capacity, available to all students and focusing on prevention. In this way, they serve as an informative resource for coping strategies or a safe location for students to use on days when they experience high levels of stress. For students in need of Tier 2 targeted prevention or intervention, the Wellness Center may be part of a plan that includes focused skill instruction for emotional regulation or daily check-ins with a trusted adult. For students requiring Tier 3 services, the Wellness Center can serve as a complement to therapy, providing reinforcement for the work done during therapy sessions or offering a de-escalation space for students who frequently require a calm environment during their school day as they are learning coping strategies.

There is evidence that students, parents, and staff perceive Wellness Centers as beneficial for mental wellness in the school environment (Moya et al., 2022). Further, research indicates that students from marginalized groups (LGBTQ+) are frequently represented in Wellness Centers (Wang et al., 2020). This is promising due to their greater risk of mental health concerns. By promoting preventative methods to decrease stress, these centers provide a touchpoint for prioritizing self-care.

They provide students with consistent access to a dedicated location for mental health and wellness services and also demonstrate a school's commitment to their overall well-being.

2.8 Summary

Tiered systems of support offer a preventive and efficient framework for delivering school mental health. Within this framework, intervention is intended to reach all students. Depending on student responsiveness, intervention intensity is systematically increased. Interventions will be most effective when procedures are established for identifying students who will receive support at each tier, while also developing a formula for moving students from tier to tier as more or less intensive supports are needed. Building and sustaining tiered supports requires organizational structure and commitment. This can be best accomplished by creating feelings of ownership, responsibility, and belongingness among all staff with leadership support. A clearly defined and operationalized system with accompanying training will facilitate this agenda. Finally, schools can capitalize on contextual features to facilitate implementation and assure the best use of resources.

References

Agyapong, B., Obuobi-Donkor, G., Burback, L., & Wei, Y. (2022). Stress, burnout, anxiety and depression among teachers: A scoping review. *International Journal of Environmental Research and Public Health, 19*(17), 10706.

American Federation of Teachers. *American Federation of Teachers*. https://www.aft.org/

Bambara, L. M., & Kern, L. (Eds.). (2021). *Individualized supports for students with problem behavior*. Paul H. Brookes.

Briesch, A. M., & Briesch, J. M. (2016). Meta-analysis of behavioral self-management interventions in single-case research. *School Psychology Review, 45*(1), 3–18.

Bruhn, A. L., Lane, K. L., & Hirsch, S. E. (2014). A review of tier 2 interventions conducted within multitiered models of behavioral prevention. *Journal of Emotional and Behavioral Disorders, 22*(3), 171–189.

CASEL. (2022). *Fundamentals of SEL*. CASEL. https://casel.org/fundamentals-of-sel/

Center for School Mental Health. (2018). *School mental health screening playbook: Best practices and tips from the field*. Retrieved from https://noys.org/sites/default/files/School-Mental-Health-Screening-Playbook.pdf

Cho Blair, K. S., Park, E. Y., & Kim, W. H. (2021). A meta-analysis of tier 2 interventions implemented within school-wide positive behavioral interventions and supports. *Psychology in the Schools, 58*(1), 141–161.

Connors, E. H., Prout, J., Vivrette, R., Padden, J., & Lever, N. (2021). Trauma-focused cognitive behavioral therapy in 13 urban public schools: Mixed methods results of barriers, facilitators, and implementation outcomes. *School Mental Health, 13*, 772–790. https://doi.org/10.1007/s12310-021-09445-7

Daily, S. M., Smith, M. L., Lilly, C. L., Davidov, D. M., Mann, M. J., & Kristjansson, A. L. (2020). Using school climate to improve attendance and grades: Understanding the importance of school satisfaction among middle and high school students. *Journal of School Health, 90*(9), 683–693. https://doi.org/10.1111/josh.12929

Dawkins, S., Tian, A. W., Newman, A., & Martin, A. (2017). Psychological ownership: A review and research agenda. *Journal of Organizational Behavior, 38*(2), 163–183.

Fletcher, J. M., & Vaughn, S. (2009). Response to intervention: Preventing and remediating academic difficulties. *Child Development Perspectives, 3*(1), 30–37.

Gee, K., Murdoch, C., Vang, T., Cuahuey, Q., & Prim, J. (2020, August). *Multi-tiered system of supports to address childhood trauma: Evidence and implications [Policy brief]*. Policy Analysis for California Education https://edpolicyinca.org/publications/multi-tiered-system-supports-address-childhood-trauma

Grove, R. D., & Hetzel, A. M. (1968). *Vital statistics rates in the United States, 1940–1960 (public health services publication 1677)*. U.S. Department of Health, Education, and Welfare.

Hawken, L. S., Crone, D. A., Bundock, K., & Horner, R. H. (2020). *Responding to problem behavior in schools*. Guilford Publications.

Hunter, K. K., Chenier, J. S., & Gresham, F. M. (2014). Evaluation of check in/check out for students with internalizing behavior problems. *Journal of Emotional and Behavioral Disorders, 22*(3), 135–148.

Jaycox, L. H., Langley, A. K., Stein, B. D., Wong, M., Sharma, P., Scott, M., & Schonlau, M. (2009). Support for students exposed to trauma: A pilot study. *School Mental Health, 1*, 49–60. https://doi.org/10.1007/s12310-009-9007-8. PMID: 20811511; PMCID: PMC2930829.

Kauer, S. D., Reid, S. C., Crooke, A. H. D., Khor, A., Hearps, S. J. C., Jorm, A. F., et al. (2012). Self-monitoring using mobile phones in the early stages of adolescent depression: Randomized controlled trial. *Journal of Medical Internet Research, 14*(3), e1858.

Kladis, K., Hawken, L. S., O'Neill, R. E., Fischer, A. J., Fuoco, K. S., O'Keeffe, B. V., & Kiuhara, S. A. (2023). Effects of check-in check-out on engagement of students demonstrating internalizing behaviors in an elementary school setting. *Behavioral Disorders, 48*(2), 83–96.

Kutcher, S., Wei, Y., McLuckie, A., & Bullock, L. (2013). Educator mental health literacy: A programme evaluation of the teacher training education on the mental health & high school curriculum guide. *Advances in School Mental Health Promotion, 6*(2), 83–93. https://doi.org/10.1080/1754730X.2013.784615

Lee, A., & Gage, N. A. (2020). Updating and expanding systematic reviews and meta-analyses on the effects of school-wide positive behavior interventions and supports. *Psychology in the Schools, 57*(5), 783–804.

Lucassen, M. F., Stasiak, K., Crengle, S., Weisz, J. R., Frampton, C. M., Bearman, S. K., Ugueto, A. M., Herren, J., Cribb-Su'a, A., Faleafa, M., Kingi-'Ulu'ave, D., Loy, J., Scott, R. M., Hartdegen, M., & Merry, S. N. (2015). Modular approach to therapy for anxiety, depression, trauma, or conduct problems in outpatient child and adolescent mental health services in New Zealand: Study protocol for a randomized controlled trial. *Trials*, (16), 457. https://doi.org/10.1186/s13063-015-0982-9. PMID: 26458917; PMCID: PMC4603305.

Marchant, M. R., Solano, B. R., Fisher, A. K., Caldarella, P., Young, K. R., & Renshaw, T. L. (2007). Modifying socially withdrawn behavior: A playground intervention for students with internalizing behaviors. *Psychology in the Schools, 44*(8), 779–794.

McLean, L., Abry, T., Taylor, M., Jimenez, M., & Granger, K. (2017). Teachers' mental health and perceptions of school climate across the transition from training to teaching. *Teaching and Teacher Education, 65*, 230–240.

Minahan, J. (2019). Trauma-informed teaching strategies. *Educational Leadership, 77*(2), 30–35.

Mitchell, B. S., Lewis, T. J., & Stormont, M. (2021). A daily check-in/check-out intervention for students with internalizing concerns. *Journal of Behavioral Education, 30*, 178–201.

Moya, M. S., Caldarella, P., Larsen, R. A., Warren, J. S., Bitton, J. R., & Feyereisen, P. M. (2022). Addressing adolescent stress in school: Perceptions of a high school wellness center. *Education and Treatment of Children, 45*(3), 277–291.

Nadeem, E., Jaycox, L. H., Langley, A. K., Wong, M., Kalaoka, S. H., & Stein, B. D. (2014). Effects of trauma on students: Early intervention through the cognitive behavioral intervention for trauma in schools. In M. D. Weist, N. A. Lever, C. P. Bradshaw, & J. Sarno Owens (Eds.), *Handbook of school mental health: Research, training, practice, and policy* (2nd ed., pp. 145–157). Springer Science + Business Media. https://doi.org/10.1007/978-1-4614-7624-5_11

NAMI: National Alliance on Mental Illness.. *NAMI: National Alliance on Mental Illness.* https://www.nami.org/

National Academies of Sciences, Engineering, and Medicine. (2023). *Addressing the long-term effects of the COVID-19 pandemic on children and families.* The National Academies Press. https://doi.org/10.17226/26809

National Center for School Mental Health (NCSMH). (2023). *School mental health quality guide: Mental health promotion services and supports (tier 1).* NCSMH, University of Maryland School of Medicine.

National School Climate Center. (2021, March 30). *What is school climate? – National School Climate Center.* https://schoolclimate.org/about/our-approach/what-is-school-climate/

Perry, Y., Petrie, K., Buckley, H., Cavanagh, L., Clarke, D., Winslade, M., et al. (2014). Effects of a classroom-based educational resource on adolescent mental health literacy: A cluster randomised controlled trial. *Journal of Adolescence, 37*(7), 1143–1151. https://doi.org/10.1016/j.adolescence.2014.08.001

Reinert, M., Fritze, D., & Nguyen, T. (2022, October). *The state of mental health in America 2023.* Mental Health America.

von der Embse, N., Ryan, S. V., Gibbs, T., & Mankin, A. (2019). Teacher stress interventions: A systematic review. *Psychology in the Schools, 56*(8), 1328–1343.

Wang, A., Tobon, J. I., Bieling, P., Jeffs, L., Colvin, E., & Zipursky, R. B. (2020). Rethinking service design for youth with mental health needs: The development of the Youth Wellness Centre, St. Joseph's Healthcare Hamilton. *Early Intervention in Psychiatry, 14*(3), 365–372.

Weist, M. D., Eber, L., Horner, R., Splett, J., Putnam, R., Barrett, S., Perales, K., Fairchild, A. J., & Hoover, S. (2018). Improving multi-tiered systems of support for students with "internalizing" emotional/behavioral problems. *Journal of Positive Behavior Interventions, 20*(3), 172–184.

Weist, M. D., Garbacz, A., Schultz, B., Bradshaw, C. P., & Lane, K. L. (2023). Revisiting the percentage of K-12 students in need of preventive interventions in schools in a "Peri-COVID" era: Implications for the implementation of tiered programming. *Prevention Science*, 1–7.

Yanek, K., Scherder, E., Haines, C., Barrett, S., Huebner, S., & Weist, M. D. (2022). Moving beyond self-care: What happens if your oxygen mask isn't dropping? *National Association of School Psychologists Communiqué, 50*(7), 1.

Zakszeski, B. N., Banks, E., & Parks, T. (2023). Targeted intervention for elementary students with internalizing behaviors: A pilot evaluation. *School Psychology Review*, 1–14. https://doi.org/10.1080/2372966X.2023.2195806

Chapter 3
Communities of Practice and Scaling Effective School Mental Health

Kristen Figas, Tucker Chandler, and Mark D. Weist

3.1 Description of Communities of Practice and Chapter Overview

When groups of people come together regularly around a shared interest, concern, or passion, a community of practice (CoP)[1] is formed (Wenger-Trayner & Wenger-Trayner, 2015; Pyrko et al., 2019). Wenger (1998) defined CoPs as "Groups of people who share a concern or a passion for something they do and learn how to do it better as they interact regularly" (p. 2). The concept of shared learning is the foundation upon which all CoPs are built, as such groups emerge to bring together a community of people who learn from and with one another. By convening regularly, members refine their knowledge and practice around a shared area of interest.

Primarily used in learning theory, the concept of CoPs can be traced back to work conducted by anthropologists Jean Lave and Etienne Wenger, who coined the term to explain the "living curriculum" through which an apprentice gains mastery over their trade (Wenger, 1998). This process is not limited to the relationship between the expert and the student but also includes learning from more seasoned apprentices (Wenger, 1998). Learning, therefore, is a dynamic process by which knowledge is passed in a way that actively shapes and is recursively shaped by its members. By naming and defining CoPs, a framework emerged that allows us to better understand this process of relationship-centered shared learning where everyone from novices to masters brings invaluable input and life to the group.

---

[1] For the purposes of this chapter, we will abbreviate community of practice as CoP and the plural communities of practice as CoPs to align with convention.

K. Figas (✉) · T. Chandler · M. D. Weist
Department of Psychology, University of South Carolina, Columbia, SC, USA
e-mail: KFIGAS@email.sc.edu; ETC3@mailbox.sc.edu; WEIST@sc.edu

We describe key elements and building CoPs at multiple levels of scale including at school building, school district, state, and regional levels. We discuss related concepts of enhancing interdisciplinary, vertical, and horizontal collaboration, present a range of challenges to CoPs in school mental health (SMH), and discuss ideas on advancing research and dissemination on this theme.

3.2 Key Elements of Communities of Practice

All CoPs are comprised of key elements that function as the basis of our understanding and identification of CoPs. These elements were conceptualized by Wenger-Trayner and Wenger-Trayner (2015) as comprising the following three elements: the domain, the community, and the practice.

3.2.1 The Domain

"The domain" refers to the shared interest, concern, or passion around which a CoP forms (Wenger-Trayner & Wenger-Trayner, 2015). The domain is the most central, integral aspect of any CoP, serving as the linchpin that connects all other elements of a CoP. The identity of a CoP is defined by this "shared domain of interest" (Wenger-Trayner & Wenger-Trayner, 2015) or "joint enterprise" of the group (Pyrko et al., 2019). Wenger-Trayner and Wenger-Trayner (2015) explained, "Membership therefore implies a commitment to the domain, and therefore a shared competence that distinguishes members from other people. The domain is not necessarily something recognized as 'expertise' outside the community" (p. 2).

3.2.2 The Community

"The community" (Wenger-Trayner & Wenger-Trayner, 2015) or "mutual engagement" (Pyrko et al., 2019) refers to the members that make up each CoP. Pyrko et al. (2019) explained membership, saying, "By engaging with other members, individuals gradually enact their membership of the community. The level of membership depends on the degree to which a person interacts meaningfully with other members and invests their identity" (p. 484). Membership is fluid and fluctuates with the ever-changing priorities and needs of the group and is also largely dependent on each member's willingness to participate and invest. Consequently, members invest at various levels based on their needs and the degree to which their participation satisfies them and aids in their learning, which allows for core and peripheral members to shift along with emerging needs (Pyrko et al., 2019).

3.2.3 The Practice

"The practice" or "shared repertoire" refers to the practices that are adopted as a result of engaging in the CoP (Pyrko et al., 2019; Wenger-Trayner & Wenger-Trayner, 2015). Pyrko et al. (2019) explained this element as "thinking together," which is when practitioners come together to share knowledge and discuss challenges specific to their shared domain. As these practitioners convene to learn from and with one another, they develop a shared repertoire of information and practices to draw upon, thus creating a way of practice that is singular to their group and much richer than their individual efforts in practice alone. Much of this is due to the tacit knowledge that each member contributes to the group, as such knowledge and practice are developed almost exclusively through experiences and cannot necessarily be taught explicitly (Pyrko et al., 2017; Polanyi, 1962). Thus, sustained learning in a social context drives practice as it allows members to draw upon others' experiences and expertise to develop skills more refined than what they can accomplish on their own (Wenger, 1998).

3.2.4 Indicators of Communities of Practice

These key elements give structure to the concept of CoPs, illuminating the core building blocks that comprise such groups. CoPs form organically as practitioners, from novices to experts, come together to address a shared topic or emergent problem relevant to their field of practice. As they draw upon each other's knowledge and experiences, they gain understanding and skills that will enhance their practice in ways that cannot be achieved alone. Aristotle's famous words capture the essence of CoPs: "The whole is greater than the sum of its parts."

Wenger's (1998) indicators of a CoP further explicate the characteristics and dynamics of the elements described above. Some of these indicators, such as sustained mutual relationships (which can be harmonious or conflictual in nature), shared ways of collaborating, and discourse around shared perspectives, describe group dynamics. Other indicators—for instance, quick setup of the problem or focus, ongoing conversation without introductory preambles, and rapid flow of information and new ideas—describe how CoPs function. Wenger (1998) also lists identity variables indicative of CoPs, including general agreement in members' definitions of who belongs to the CoP; understanding other members' knowledge base, skills, and potential contributions; recognizing certain styles as indicating membership in the CoP; and members engaging in a process of mutually defining identities. The remaining indicators describe processes and outcomes that characterize CoPs, such as the ability to evaluate actions and products, specific tools and resources, local lore and shared narratives, and jargon and communication shortcuts to facilitate conversation. These indicators lay the foundation for effective convening: gathering the right people together; creating a climate for participant genuine engagement; and moving from discussion to dialogue, to collaboration and mutual support, and ultimately to positive policy change and resource enhancement (see Cashman et al., 2014).

3.3   Organic Nature of Communities of Practice

Learning cannot be designed. Ultimately, it belongs to the realm of experience and practice. It follows the negotiation of meaning; it moves on its own terms. It slips through the cracks; it creates its own cracks. Learning happens, design or no design. And yet there are few more urgent tasks than to design social infrastructures that foster learning (Wenger, 1998, p. 225).

It is vital to note that one of the most distinguishing qualities of CoPs is their inherent ambiguity and fluidity. Wenger-Trayner and Wenger-Trayner (2015) explains that this conceptualization, "Allows for, but does not assume, intentionality: learning can be the reason the community comes together or an incidental outcome of member's interactions. Not everything called a community is a community of practice. A neighborhood for instance, is often called a community, but is usually not a community of practice" (p. 2). Recognizing the imprecision of CoPs is critical for understanding both what they are and what they are not. While many groups come together to learn, even to learn from and with one another, CoPs are distinguished by their organic emergence and evolution, arising to meet the specific needs of a particular group of people at a particular time. This process of fluid formation and constant evolution is the key ingredient that gives CoPs their potential for influence, impact, and meaning, as both problems and membership continually shift to meet the emerging needs of the larger community.

Although CoPs hinge on non-hierarchical dynamics, shared ownership, and collaborative co-learning, leadership still plays a pivotal role. Committed and sustained leadership is imperative to growing and maintaining CoPs. Indeed, leadership is a significant predictor of CoP effectiveness, people's satisfaction with them, and impact on the work involved (Hemmasi & Csanda, 2009). Leaders steer the learning agenda by ensuring relevance to the domain (although members often help define the domain), attending to social dynamics and managing conflict, ensuring time is well used, documenting insights and products, and facilitating external communication (Wenger-Trayner et al., 2022). The fundamental goal of leaders is to provide the structure and opportunity for peer-to-peer learning to occur. Thus, they take on the role of a facilitator and might suggest a structure or activities to promote peer-to-peer learning, although they do not direct that learning. The challenge to leaders is that their leadership role within CoPs requires them to play a consequential behind-the-scenes role while refraining from directing the conversations and leading the learning that occurs in the CoP. This shift in dynamic may be foreign to some leaders and members alike but is vital to developing and maintaining school-level CoPs.

Inevitably, CoPs form within and across organizations and systems as individuals and groups make connections. These connections do not rely on formal structures but are emergent, with interconnections and group cohesion emerging over time. As Pyrko et al. (2019) stated, "The role of managers is increasingly regarded as not being about control, but about cultivating working environments where people are engaged, and where they trust and care for each other. CoPs are promoted as being of value to the organization so that employees' discretionary space increases and so they can take the responsibility for their learning and for their practice in their own hands" (p. 495).

3.4 Building Communities of Practice to Advance Scaling of Effective School Mental Health

In their guidebook, Wenger-Trayner et al. (2022) delineate key organizational factors, processes, and strategies for establishing and sustaining CoPs. They highlight two organizational structures undergirding CoPs: sponsors and the social learning team. There are multiple types of sponsors—initiative, domain, local, and individual—each with its own unique characteristics and goals. Initiative sponsors are often high-level executives or a leadership team (social, emotional, behavioral, and mental health [SEBMH] lead team) whose aim is to legitimize and sustain the CoP; their work is external to the CoP itself. Domain sponsors are managers who understand the significance of the CoP's domain; they engage with CoP members without controlling CoP dynamics and advocate to initiative sponsors and others about the importance of the CoP. Local sponsors are intermediate managers who encourage local participation in the CoP. Finally, individual sponsors are often direct supervisors of the constituents of the CoP; their primary goal is to ensure that the CoP is recognized as a worthwhile and valuable part of CoP members' work. When building a CoP, it is critical to identify sponsors who can use their influence to promote the CoP at each level. Whereas sponsors promote the CoP, the social learning team runs the CoP. This team leads the initiative, educates and trains leaders to develop community engagement, and addresses logistical issues (Wenger-Trayner et al., 2022). Wenger-Trayner et al. (2022) recommend attending to visibility early on (e.g., having a structure for new members to join and promoting the CoP at fairs, conferences, and summits) and being intentional with capacity building efforts, which might include building relationships with potential CoP sponsors, training community leaders and facilitators, and connecting leaders across relevant CoPs.

Understanding readiness for a CoP can help tailor capacity building efforts for optimal impact (see Splett et al., 2022). CoPs can be regarded as innovations and analyzed using existing readiness frameworks. For instance, using the $R = MC^2$ framework, involving R for readiness, M for motivation, and C^2 for general and innovation-specific organizational capacity (Scaccia et al., 2015), the social learning team might examine their and others' motivation for the CoP, considering to what extent the CoP seems more useful than alternatives (e.g., workshops and webinar, coaching, professional mentorship programs, online discussion forums), aligns with existing efforts, is easy to use and trial, has observable benefits, and is a priority. This can be supplemented with other attitudinal indicators of CoP readiness, such as a desire to improve strategic thinking, readiness for leaders to relinquish control and welcome staff leadership, valuing continuous learning, investment in work, and commitment to free up members' time to participate (Wenger-Trayner et al., 2022). Developing innovation-specific capacity (Scaccia et al., 2015) should include equipping leaders and members with the knowledge and skills to implement and participate in the CoP, identifying champions to advocate for the CoP, fostering a supportive climate with the necessary resources to promote the CoP, and developing intra- and inter- organizational relationships to encourage participation in the CoP. Finally, the social learning team should facilitate the development of general capacity (Scaccia et al., 2015), which might include developing norms and values about learning; fostering connectedness and openness to change; improving internal operations and resource utilization; promoting leadership development; advocating for sufficient staffing; and supporting planning, implementation, and evaluation.

3.4.1   Building Interdisciplinary Collaboration

Interdisciplinary collaboration is integral to the success of CoPs and to the effectiveness of SMH programs as collaborative relationships represent important social capital and serve as the foundation for systematic work (Mellin & Weist, 2011; Waxman et al., 1999). Because CoPs exist at multiple levels of scale, best practices in building interdisciplinary collaboration should be considered at both the vertical and horizontal levels. Vertical collaboration refers to the relationships between individuals and groups at multiple levels, like a school building and school district. Horizontal collaboration refers to the relationship between individuals and groups at the same level, such as a partnership between a school-based clinician and a teacher. Interdisciplinary collaboration across CoPs is illustrated through the concepts of constellations of practices (Wenger, 1998) and landscapes of practice (Pyrko et al., 2019), which are the larger bodies of practice that encompass smaller CoPs with similar and related interests. These groups include all practitioners within a specific area and promote interdisciplinary collaboration as members of related CoPs transfer knowledge and ultimately develop competence across boundaries.

3.4.2   Building Vertical Collaboration

Strong vertical collaboration is a vital component of successful CoPs, and leaders at each level play a crucial role in creating and sustaining this potential for collaboration. Leaders at higher levels (district, state, regional) nurture vertical relationships by incorporating lessons learned from smaller scales (in and across schools and districts) into decision-making and resource allocation. This not only strengthens relationships between leaders and personnel across vertical boundaries but also ensures that key voices from each level contribute to the decisions that impact their daily work. Where vertical collaboration is prioritized, shared learning becomes both a practice and a tool that strengthens the entire system.

3.4.3   Building Horizontal Collaboration

Horizontal collaboration is at the heart of every CoP, as it shapes, guides, and sustains their practice and existence. Horizontal collaboration drives shared learning among members of CoPs, providing a structure within which knowledge is transferred and skills are refined. While strong vertical collaboration can certainly set a strong foundation in which CoPs can grow and thrive, the very nature of CoPs relies on peer-to-peer learning and problem-solving to emerge from its members rather than its leaders. By collaborating with staff at the same level to build skills and tackle relevant challenges, members of CoPs control the pace and direction of the group. This not only provides strong professional development through peer-to-peer learning but also allows CoPs to evolve based on the needs and ideas of their members.

3.5   Building Communities of Practice at Multiple Levels of Scale in School Mental Health

In the following sections, we briefly review the development of SMH CoPs at multiple levels of scale including, school building, district, state, and regional levels. Please see Weist et al. (2022) for more detailed discussion of CoPs at these levels focused on the implementation of effective SMH programming.

3.5.1   Building Communities of Practice at the School Level

CoPs form at the school-building level when individuals come together around a shared interest, concern, or passion, and may have a more targeted purpose than those at broader levels. Interdisciplinary collaboration at the school level is generally focused on enhancing knowledge and developing skills that practitioners use in their everyday work (Pyrko et al., 2019), with activities relating to problem-solving and developing skills for specific tasks, projects, and roles. For example, a CoP at the school level might discuss the continuum of services provided within the school's MTSS, the options for interventions across tiers, data collection and data-informed decision-making, collaboration with other school staff, and how to support implementation of various initiatives and programs within the building. CoPs at the school level likely involve building-level staff, families and caregivers, and members of the community who all share a mutual interest in investing in the success and well-being of their students and children. School-level CoPs provide opportunities for individuals across roles to connect (e.g., teachers, clinicians, specialists, family members, and community agency providers) or may be limited to a particular subset (e.g., only teachers). These CoPs are analogous to professional learning communities (PLCs), in which teachers convene in a more structured format for peer-to-peer learning and problem-solving (Olivier & Huffman, 2016), with interdisciplinary members and a less formal structure.

Notably, a critical aspect of school-level CoPs is teaming. School-level CoPs operate alongside school teams and share similar attributes, such as bringing together multiple individuals to share expertise in pursuit of a common goal. However, team functioning in schools is commonly problematic, with many different teams, overlaps in their functioning, poor use of data, inconsistent agendas and poor follow-up (Splett et al., 2024). While many schools and SMH leaders advocate for multiple teams within the schools' MTSS (e.g., one each focusing on Tier 1, 2, and 3), our view is that a key strategy is for schools to choose one team (e.g., the SEBMH lead team) that will focus on programming across tiers related to students' social, emotional, behavioral, and mental health functioning. This avoids logistical issues of convening multiple teams, and the fragmentation that can occur with different teams meeting about what should be a unified agenda, aligned across tiers for implementing strategies that promote mental health, wellness, and school success and respond to mental health challenges. This team should be inclusive of the key staff with a vested interest in the work (e.g., school administrator, school-and community-employed mental health staff, educators, school health staff, family members), meet consistently on-time with well-established agendas, and have strong follow-up to decisions made at team meetings (Splett et al., 2024).

School-level CoPs can support the work of school teams by bolstering each team member's knowledge and skills related to their area of expertise, which can then be shared and leveraged in team meetings. For instance, the student support team[2] might only have one or two teacher representatives; by participating in a school-level CoP with other teachers, these representatives can hone skills and develop a common discourse with other teachers on SMH concerns, which they can then bring to the student support team. In this way, individual members can act as liaisons between school teams and school-level CoPs, hastening the transfer of knowledge and skills within the school community. That said, school-level CoPs are likely vulnerable to the same challenges as school teams and thus might be strengthened

---

[2] A student support team—alternatively known as a student assistance team; MTSS team; Tier 1, Tier 2, or Tier 3 team; or problem solving team—is a group of educators, staff, and, when appropriate, caregivers who collaboratively examine data to identify student concerns and match students to appropriate programs and interventions.

by attending to some of the same factors listed above (e.g., membership, consistency of meetings, and accountability for action).

School leaders play a pivotal role in promoting school-level CoPs. Principals and other leaders can enhance staff motivation and buy-in by linking CoPs to existing professional learning initiatives and school goals and communicating that CoPs are a worthwhile activity for staff. However, supportive attitudes are insufficient without accompanying structural changes that support the CoP. School leaders can allocate time for members to participate in the CoP and provide support (e.g., substitutes) to promote participation. School leaders also play an important role in building general capacity within their school. For instance, they can catalyze change in norms and values that support CoPs, conveying that they value this form of learning, and engage in community-building within their school and the local community to strengthen networks outside of the CoP. In this way, school leaders can also promote the natural development of CoPs outside of those formally championed. Of course, school leaders also answer to the district, and educators and the local community respond to values and norms conveyed by the district, making district buy-in and support essential to school-level CoPs.

3.5.2 Building Communities of Practice at the District Level

At the district level, SMH CoPs likely have a different purpose than those at the school level. For instance, they might be focused on learning about how to best support implementation of SMH, improving SEBMH/SMH teaming or data practices, or building SMH resources district-wide. As reviewed earlier, membership of CoPs therefore should extend beyond district and school employees and should include community members such as families and caregivers, youth-serving systems (education, mental health, child welfare, juvenile justice, primary health care, disabilities) as well as faith and business leaders. There may be multiple district-level CoPs supporting effective SMH, with some connecting individuals with like-roles across the district, and others connecting individuals with varied roles. Each of these may or may not include vertical collaboration (e.g., including supervisors, directors, and other leaders). Vertical collaboration (down to buildings and back up) is particularly important in district-level CoPs, as on-the-ground perspectives should inform district decision-making.

Developing district-level CoPs requires fostering relationships within the district and surrounding community, promoting norms and values that increase buy-in, enacting structural changes and allocating resources to support CoPs, and developing mechanisms for supporting CoP implementation. Building capacity for collaboration and shared learning across the district and community might include novel approaches for engaging with community members to strengthen the partnerships and networks that underlie the CoP. This might include strengthening existing partnership and teaming structures to ensure district employees and community members have voice in district decision-making. Members' voice can also be used to inform the structure, format, and frequency of meetings of district CoPs.

Changing norms and values and securing buy-in becomes more complicated at this scale; however, there are more opportunities at the district level to create structures that support CoPs, which in turn communicate the norm shift to individuals in the schools. For instance, dedicating time to participate in CoPs may require changes to how professional development is structured and/or scheduled. Adjusting traditional professional development options with opportunities to participate in CoPs would strongly communicate the district's investment in this form of learning and build readiness. Additionally, districts might offer incentives (e.g., compensation, extra personal days, or other enticements) to motivate participation, especially early on.

District teams also play an important role in strengthening general capacity by investing in leadership development and equipping members with the knowledge and skills (e.g., training and coaching leaders and members on CoP practices) to promote collaborative and productive CoPs at both the district and school levels. This might include hiring specialists and coaches to support implementation of CoPs and establishing processes for accessing support.

The Interconnected Systems Framework for Positive Behavioral Interventions and Supports (PBIS) and SMH emphasizes the critical role of district-community leadership teams (DCLT) that organize to coordinate programming district-wide and to support effective implementation of SMH interventions at school building levels across Tier 1 (prevention), Tier 2 (early intervention), and Tier 3 (more intensive intervention) of schools' multitiered systems of support (MTSS; Eber et al., 2020; Chap. 2, this volume).

3.5.3   Building Communities of Practice at the State Level

At the state level, SMH CoPs may be oriented toward more macrosystemic change, such as building infrastructure that supports effective SMH in schools and advocating for funding and policy change. State-level CoPs may take many forms, existing concurrently in the same domain while pursuing different goals. Some state-level CoPs may have larger and/or more diverse membership than school- and district-level CoPs, although others may be more contained. Representatives from the state department of education, state department of mental health, and policymakers might be included in these CoPs, alongside school-level educators and practitioners, community and school mental health clinicians, school and district leaders, and other youth-serving systems and organizations (e.g., health care, social services, juvenile justice, positive youth development, family advocacy). Some state-level CoPs might include members from a combination of these communities, whereas others might convene individuals occupying the same role across the state (e.g., all school counselors). Membership boundaries and meeting structure and format for state-level CoPs likely vary depending on the purpose of the CoP. Some CoPs might engage exclusively in horizontal collaboration, for example, enabling representations from different state departments to learn from one another and tailor and/or build upon existing systems and supports instead of starting anew. Although all state-level CoPs need not include vertical collaboration, this is important to incorporate to some degree to hasten knowledge transfer and use local evidence to inform state-level SMH initiatives.

At the state level, CoPs may focus on building infrastructure that supports implementation, policy, funding mechanisms, dissemination of best practices, and development of standards. District, state, and regional leaders are involved at this level as well as various constituents, organizations, and systems with vested interests. As in district-community leadership teams, state-level CoPs should include leaders from all youth-serving systems with a vested interest in SMH, including education, mental health, child welfare, juvenile justice, primary care, and disabilities systems, along with community leaders such as business and faith leaders.

Leaders of state licensing bodies, state agencies, and state professional organizations (e.g., state association of school social workers) can publicize CoPs to their constituents. State leaders can also influence norms through guidance disseminated to districts and schools, legitimizing CoPs and encouraging participation. State departments and organizations can develop manuals and other informational materials and coordinate training and technical assistance for CoPs to facilitate their implementation. State departments of education and/or mental health can also invest in developing infrastructure that supports implementation of CoPs and helps members and leaders adapt to local context. This should include training, coaching, and technical assistance and might include workshops, clinics, or demonstrations to increase awareness and understanding of CoPs.

3.5.4 Building Communities of Practice at the Regional Level

Regional CoPs and similar initiatives can strengthen capacity for SMH CoPs across levels. Regional networks bring together individuals at various levels across multiple states. For instance, these networks might include educators, school specialists, school leaders, mental health clinicians, state representatives and policymakers, community members, and researchers, among others to share perspectives, opportunities, and initiatives on school mental health. By fostering connections across states and diversifying the contexts, resources, and perspectives represented by members, these networks are ripe for creative problem-solving and vast dissemination of knowledge.

Regional CoPs may form across school, district, and state boundaries to encompass a larger community focused on addressing challenges and promoting best practices within the field. For example, the Southeastern School Behavioral Health Community (SSBHC, see www.schoolbehavioralhealth.org) includes 12 states sharing experiences and lessons learned in bringing effective SMH practices to scale. The SSBHC is organized in South Carolina and includes state advisors from the 11 other southeastern states who meet virtually throughout the year and once during a preconference focusing on effective SMH. The most recent (April 2023) SSBHC conference included 1000 participants (700 in-person, 300 virtual), with growth expected for this CoP and conference in the years to come.

There are also regional CoPs supporting effective MTSS/PBIS in schools including networks in the Mid-Atlantic (www.midatlanticpbis.org), Midwest (www.midwestpbis.org), Northeast (www.northeastpbis.org), and Northwest (www.northwestpbis.org). Of note, leaders from these regional CoPs focused on the advancement of school mental health and MTSS often convene together at national conferences, including meetings of the Council for Exceptional Children (www.cec.org), PBIS National Leadership Forum (www.pbis.org), and National Center for School Mental Health (www.schoolmentalhealth.org). Knowledge exchanged by regional leaders at these national meetings in turn informs work occurring at state, district, and school building levels, collectively escalating the pace of positive change for the field.

Strong examples of regional CoPs can serve as exemplars, demonstrating how to establish connections and link existing networks. For example, the Carolina Network for School Mental Health is a network of K-12 educators, academics, mental health professionals, and school, district, and state leaders that aims to facilitate collaborations across North and South Carolina to expand access to effective youth mental health promotion, prevention, and intervention services (see www.carolinanetwork.org). The Carolina Network meets in person annually and has endured for more than a decade, gaining new members each year. At meetings, members form new connections, share information about SMH initiatives in each state, identify challenges and discuss possible solutions, and develop research-practice partnerships. Thus, regional initiatives like the SSBHC and Carolina Network can create and strengthen professional connections in service of disseminating best practices, propelling state-level change, and informing both research and practice.

3.6 Challenges to Building Communities of Practice

Communities of practice can be challenging to establish and sustain. Wenger-Trayner et al. (2022) enumerated foreseeable barriers to CoPs in their recently published guidebook. The authors caution that the popularity of CoPs can contribute to CoPs becoming a fad concept, resulting in misapplication of the term (Wenger-Trayner et al., 2022). Other challenges include perfunctory participation and micromanagement, which interferes with members developing a sense of ownership and undermines collaboration and learning. Adhering to a restrictive agenda and being overly task-oriented can be perceived as burdensome and have a similarly limiting effect. On the other hand, internal politics, including fluctuations in leadership, attitudes, and priorities, and organizational neglect pose challenges for sustaining CoPs.

Additionally, dynamics within CoPs can limit their effect and threaten their growth and development. For instance, CoPs can become insular when members are singularly focused on a topic and/or establish rigid boundaries for membership, limiting the flow of new perspectives (Wenger-Trayner et al., 2022). CoPs are vulnerable to problematic groupthink, the domination of a few voices, discontinuity across meetings, and reliance on didactic presentations over discussion. There is also a risk that leaders will regard the CoP as a service for members (as opposed to a co-learning environment) or a project for which the leaders are responsible, which can impede the development of shared ownership and peer-to-peer learning.

3.7 Challenges to Building Communities of Practice in School Mental Health

SMH presents a number of unique challenges stemming from service fragmentation, resource constraints, diverse perspectives and priorities, and underdeveloped infrastructure and foundational practices. This is also related to the fact that effective SMH involves cross-system partnerships (primarily education and mental health systems, but other systems as reviewed earlier). Thus, SMH leaders need to navigate culture and policies and procedures for each system, as well as those developed specifically for the cross-system collaboration (e.g., memoranda of agreement between schools and community mental health agencies. A recent handbook on SMH (Evans et al., 2023) provides a deeper review of these and other issues.

3.7.1 Service Fragmentation

Fueled by federalism's dispersion of power (states' rights, local control), SMH policies and practices differ markedly between states as well as across districts within a state (National Center for School Mental Health, 2023). Similarly, educational and mental health infrastructure, funding, licensure/certification, and approaches to continuing education vary by state. Districts are given local control to determine how to actualize policies and allocate funds, resulting in varied approaches to supporting students' well-being. This variability can impede the development and work of CoPs in multiple ways. For instance, when individuals with the same professional role have different responsibilities across districts, it can complicate the effort to identify and link individuals working to strengthen SMH programming. Differences in contexts, resources, and approaches across schools can distract members from a common goal or stoke a dynamic that laments barriers without identifying solutions. Divergent perspectives and priorities of school and district leaders can also interfere with CoPs, opening or closing opportunities to form or participate in CoPs. Site-based management of schools can exacerbate this variability and limit scaling; for example, there is wide variability in principal support for the social, emotional, behavioral, mental health agenda in schools, with some principals making almost exclusive emphasis on the academic performance of students (see Lyon et al., 2018).

3.7.2 Resource Constraints and Conflicting Priorities

Chronic resource constraints in the educational and mental health systems and the associated competition of priorities can similarly hinder CoPs. In particular, inadequate funding and staffing limit the availability of mental and behavioral health programs, supports, and services in schools (Panchal et al., 2022). Academic initiatives, whether curricula and interventions for students or professional development for teachers, often outcompete SMH initiatives, contributing to inertia in developing CoPs focused on SMH. Inadequate resources might also lead to CoPs being implemented haphazardly and/or incorrectly, with ramifications for effectiveness and sustainability.

CoPs may be deprioritized when they collide with traditional approaches to continuing learning (e.g., didactic professional development). Many educators are accustomed to hierarchical leadership structures and expert-driven training, which may lead to initial discomfort with the collaborative, co-learning dynamic of CoPs. Likewise, districts might view CoPs as conflicting with existing professional development structures or be reluctant to relinquish control over training by incorporating non-hierarchical, peer-to-peer approaches to professional learning. Moreover, educators and SMH professionals are bound by existing continuing education systems to maintain licensure and/or certification, and participating in CoPs may conflict with other learning opportunities that offer needed credits.

3.7.3 Underdeveloped Data Systems and Practices

Underdeveloped data systems and practices pose yet another challenge to SMH CoPs. Schools have been slow to roll out universal mental health screening (Burns & Rapee, 2022; Connors et al., 2022; Wood & McDaniel, 2022). The most common barriers to conducting SMH screening stem from resource constraints (lack of time and personnel resources), followed by worries about follow-up, lack of knowledge, and the cost (Burns & Rapee, 2022; Splett et al., 2018). This points to underdeveloped infrastructure, knowledge, and skills for collecting, managing, analyzing, and using mental health data in schools. Critically, this suggests that data are not being widely used to inform decisions about SMH. This presents a significant hurdle for SMH interventions and supports, including CoPs, as the absence of foundational data practices in place complicates the tasks of justifying and evaluating school mental health CoPs.

Fragmentation, limited resources, conflicting priorities, and underdeveloped data practices create unique challenges to establishing and sustaining CoPs in

SMH. Highly variable programming and practices across schools, districts, and states, combined with chronic resource shortages, highlight the need to move toward more uniform and lower cost approaches to measurement and programming. Making measures and programs publicly available will promote interdisciplinary collaboration within CoPs by equalizing access to resources and removing a significant barrier to knowledge transfer. As programs become more available and are increasingly disseminated through CoPs, it is important that this situation is met with a complementary effort to de-implement programs or practices that are ineffective or a poor fit, in order to alleviate unnecessary strain and confusion (see Eber et al., 2020). CoPs might also provide the support members need to identify candidate programs and practices and move toward de-implementation. In this way, CoPs can be leveraged to reduce fragmentation, overcome some resource constraints, and improve systemic decision-making, mitigating the very barriers to their development and ultimately strengthening capacity for SMH.

3.8 Building the Research Agenda on Communities of Practice in School Mental Health

To build forward momentum, it is critical that efforts to build and expand CoPs are met with a defined research agenda focused on strengthening the concept, evaluating outcomes, and examining influential variables and mechanisms of action.

3.8.1 Strengthening the Concept

Drawing conclusions about the effectiveness of CoPs and understanding how effects are attained is predicated on having a clear and consistent definition of the concept. While Wenger's (1998) three key elements (e.g., domain, community, practice) and other indicators provide conceptual parameters for CoPs, they lack specificity, muddying the boundaries between CoPs and similar concepts (e.g., professional learning communities, learning collaboratives, professional networks). Efforts to operationalize CoP elements and processes will enhance the utility of the term and enable the growth of a knowledge base explicitly pertaining to CoPs. This should include identifying core and peripheral elements, key structures and processes, including how CoPs develop and interact (Pyrko et al., 2017; Pyrko et al., 2019). Other avenues include better understanding interpersonal and power dynamics of CoPs and the role and characteristics of CoP leaders (Bootz et al., 2023; Pyrko et al., 2019; Roberts, 2006). This effort to improve operational specificity of CoPs should be accompanied by the development of standardized measures and tools that can be used in research and practical applications to build and evaluate CoPs (Lardier et al., 2023).

Once the base concept is operationalized, researchers can explore variations, such as strategic enhancements. For instance, does incorporating more systematic problem-solving approaches improve outcomes, as suggested by Barbour et al. (2018)? Although some may argue this veers from the essence of a CoP, following a more structured problem-solving process, such as the team-initiated problem-solving (TIPS) framework (Newton et al., 2009) or action circles (Action Circles, 2022) may offer added benefits. Both approaches are goal-oriented and provide a structure for identifying solutions, enacting change, and evaluating progress. Overlaying this structure on a CoP might focus conversations and foster a productive dynamic, while still allowing members to drive the process and learn from one another, with the added benefit of helping to further operationalize the concept.

3.8.2 Evaluating Impact

Evaluating the impact of CoPs is an underdeveloped area of study, with most empirical research being very recent. Efforts to evaluate CoPs are hampered by poor measurement options (Lardier et al., 2023), as well as lack of consensus over the relevant dependent variables. Thus, defining dependent variables of interest and developing valid and reliable measurement tools are critical steps.

Wenger-Trayner et al. (2022) recommend focusing on engagement and perceived value as metrics of success. Recent research offers multiple examples of how these outcomes might be examined. For example, Giebel et al. (2023) evaluated engagement, experiences, and perceived impact of a CoP on dementia research using mixed methods, finding that the CoP increased participants' research capacity and knowledge, improved connections between constituents, and improved access to care. Other research teams have examined perceived impact and value of CoPs for special educators (Hirsch et al., 2023) and mental consultants (Seguin et al., 2023), examining stress/emotional exhaustion, perceived value, and perceived benefits to professional practice as dependent variables. Hirsch et al. (2023) found that participants perceived the CoP as beneficial despite obtaining null results for stress and emotional exhaustion. However, the CoP in this study was relatively brief (four 60-minute meetings), which raises the question of how much engagement or participation is needed to derive measurable benefits.

SMH CoPs might include outcomes beyond those listed above. For instance, SMH CoPs might impact teacher, clinician, and leader variables, such as improving knowledge, attitudes, and skills, enhancing self-efficacy, and reducing burnout. Findings from a CoP focused on preventing youth substance use (Anderson-Carpenter et al., 2014) suggest that SMH CoPs might also impact systemic variables like enhancing partnerships and implementation of evidence-based practices across communities. Through their impact on these proximal outcomes, SMH CoPs, especially those at the school and district level, might also be associated with changes in more distal outcomes, such as student social-emotional-behavioral and mental health functioning, and school climate.

3.8.3 Exploring Moderators and Mediators

Strengthening the concept and evaluating outcomes allow for the examination of moderating variables that strengthen or attenuate the relationship between CoPs and outcomes of interest. In other words, for whom and under what circumstances are SMH CoPs effective? Abedini et al. (2021) identified a number of characteristics of CoP members, including being independent, experience- and problem-centered, self-motivated, goal-oriented, and committed to lifelong learning. Although these characteristics were not empirically examined as moderators, different degrees of these or other characteristics might influence the benefits derived from a CoP. Similarly, leadership styles, characteristics, and activities might be more aligned with some CoPs than others (Bootz et al., 2023; Hemmasi & Csanda, 2009), possibly moderating the impact of the CoP on outcomes. Other factors like staff burnout, trust, connectedness, and the level of engagement/participation might alter the impact CoPs have on outcomes (Abedini et al., 2021; Hemmasi & Csanda, 2009; Lardier et al., 2023).

Alongside investigating moderators, it is important to examine mediating variables to elucidate mechanisms of action through which SMH CoPs impact outcomes. For instance, CoPs might lead to teams adopting innovative strategies, which results in improvements in SMH programming. CoPs might also help members identify strategies that promote implementation, thus improving the acceptability, feasibility, fidelity, and sustainability of initiatives. Members might also learn new approaches to partnering with mental health providers, increasing the availability of SMH services. Changes in accessibility, quality, and implementation of SMH services, in turn, may lead to change in student outcomes.

3.8.4 Developing Conceptual Frameworks

Empirical research on CoPs is still in the early stages, and there are many avenues for advancing this body of knowledge. Figure 3.1 summarizes these opportunities in a conceptual framework for conducting research on SMH CoPs. The elements included in the framework represent some of the key features, processes, and outcomes delineated in this chapter but are far from exhaustive. This conceptual framework can and likely will change as the body of research on SMH CoPs expands and identifies new avenues and priorities.

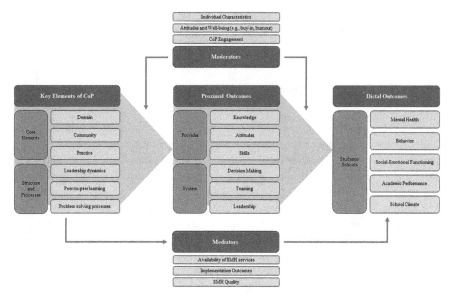

Fig. 3.1 CoP conceptual framework

3.9 Disseminating Communities of Practice to Advance Their Scaling in School Mental Health

The imprecision of the concept and early stage of research on CoPs underscore the need to develop and publicize strong model demonstration programs to provide members, leaders, and sponsors with a vision of what SMH CoPs might look like. While model CoPs are being developed, strategies for disseminating these exemplars should also be explored. These strategies should be tailored to desired audiences to build awareness across the many professional roles that may be represented in SMH CoPs. A combination of traditional and innovative strategies may be most effective.

3.9.1 Traditional Dissemination

Traditional mechanisms like publications, presentations, site visits, and listservs can build awareness of CoPs in the scientific and practice communities. Publication should include a variety of products (e.g., peer-reviewed manuscripts, books and chapters, manuals, and guidance documents) geared toward multiple consumer groups (e.g., academics, educators, practitioners, leaders, and family and youth advocates). Ensuring most products are freely available and easily accessible will help to advance dissemination efforts. Presenting successful examples at conferences, summits, and professional meetings in both the education and mental health fields, as well as offering on-site tours that include opportunities to meet individuals working to build CoPs (such as at colleges and universities, regional centers, and state departments), may ignite interest and secure buy-in. Using existing networks and infrastructure to share information through listservs and newsletters may reach individuals overlooked by other dissemination mechanisms.

3.9.2 Innovative Dissemination

These more traditional approaches could be supplemented with innovative approaches that utilize preferred technology to reach potential members. This might include broader marketing campaigns using the principles of social marketing and strategically leveraging social media. Such marketing campaigns might utilize different social network sites to share information about and examples of CoPs to specific audiences (e.g., sharing with academics on X [formerly, Twitter], and using Facebook and Instagram to target educational, mental health, and other communities). Offering live or recorded virtual, or virtual reality, demonstrations or clinics that provide opportunities for individuals to observe or "try out" CoPs may also generate engagement and help reach individuals who are unable to attend in-person events but prefer a more interactive experience.

Other innovative approaches that nurture communities while promoting knowledge sharing and mutual support can be used to both build and disseminate CoPs. For example, the Extension for Community Healthcare Outcomes (ECHO) model (Project ECHO, n.d.) provides a structure for developing virtual CoPs that unite individuals with varying levels of expertise around a common goal and emphasize multidirectional, peer-to-peer learning (Struminger et al., 2017). The ECHO model fosters the key elements of CoPs while overcoming several shortcomings through better specified operating procedures and infrastructure for training and implementation support. The ECHO website (https://projectecho.unm.edu) also offers tools for searching and joining existing ECHOs and starting a new ECHO, simultaneously expanding established CoPs and cultivating new ones.

3.10 Conclusion

Communities of practice can serve as strong platforms for enhancing current and ongoing efforts in SMH at all levels of practice, offering both structure and opportunity for those with vested interests to convene around shared problems and spark change. Key considerations for developing and strengthening such groups include identifying the unique challenges for each group and highlighting and building upon the strengths and opportunities singular to each community. Other considerations include securing buy-in from members, evaluating readiness, defining purpose, and establishing connections across CoPs to ensure each CoP truly reflects the nature of the community involved and meets the specific needs they are seeking to meet.

Acknowledgments We thank Sarah Dremann, Esperanza Lopez, and Stacy Phillips for their help in reviewing relevant literature for this chapter.

References

Abedini, A., Abedin, B., & Zowghi, D. (2021). Adult learning in online communities of practice: A systematic review. *British Journal of Educational Technology, 52*, 1663–1694. https://doi.org/10.1111/bjet.13120

Action circles. (2022). *Values to action: Social justice for everyone's well-being.* Retrieved December 20, 2023 from https://www.valuestoaction.org/actioncircles

Anderson-Carpenter, K. D., Watson-Thompson, J., Jones, M., & Chaney, L. (2014). Using communities of practice to support implementation of evidence-based prevention strategies. *Journal of Community Practice, 22*(1–2), 176–188. https://doi.org/10.1080/10705422.2014.901268

Barbour, L., Armstrong, R., Condron, P., & Palermo, C. (2018). Communities of practice to improve public health outcomes: A systematic review. *Journal of Knowledge Management, 22*(2), 326–343. https://doi.org/10.1108/JKM-03-2017-0111

Bootz, J., Borzillo, S., & Raub, S. (2023). Leaders of organisational communities of practice: Their characteristics, activities, and fit with their communities. *Knowledge Management Research & Practice, 21*(5), 972–982. https://doi.org/10.1080/14778238.2022.2120837

Burns, J. R., & Rapee, R. M. (2022). Barriers to universal mental health screening in schools: The perspective of school psychologists. *Journal of Applied School Psychology, 38*(3), 223–240. https://doi.org/10.1080/15377903.2021.1941470

Cashman, J., Linehan, P., Purcell, L., Rosser, M., Schultz, S., & Skalski, S. (2014). *Leading by convening: A blueprint for authentic engagement.* National Association of State Directors of Special Education.

Connors, E. H., Moffa, K., Carter, T., Crocker, J., Bohnenkamp, J. H., Lever, N. A., & Hoover, S. A. (2022). Advancing mental health screening in schools: Innovative, field-tested practices and observed trends during a 15-month learning collaborative. *Psychology in the Schools, 59*(6), 1135–1157. https://doi.org/10.1002/pits.22670

Eber, L., Barrett, S., Perales, K., Jeffrey-Pearsall, J., Pohlman, K., Putnam, R., Splett, J., & Weist, M. D. (2020). *Advancing education effectiveness: Interconnecting school mental health and school-wide PBIS, Volume 2: An implementation guide.* Center for Positive Behavioral Interventions and Supports (funded by the Office of Special Education Programs, U.S. Department of Education). Eugene, Oregon: University of Oregon Press.

Evans, S. W., Owens, J. S., Bradshaw, C. P., & Weist, M. D. (2023). *Handbook of school mental health: Innovations in science and practice* (3rd ed.). Springer.

Giebel, C., Tetlow, H., Faulkner, T., & Eley, R. (2023). A community of practice to increase education and collaboration in dementia and ageing research and care: The Liverpool dementia & ageing research forum. *Health Expectations, 26*, 1977–1985. https://doi.org/10.1111/hex.13806

Hemmasi, M., & Csanda, C. M. (2009). The effectiveness of communities of practice: An empirical study. *Journal of Managerial Issues, 21*(2), 262–279.

Hirsch, S. E., Mathews, H. M., Griffith, C., Carlson, A., & Walker, A. (2023). Fostering social support and professional learning for special educators: Building a community of practice. *Journal of Emotional and Behavioral Disorders, 31*(2), 132–143. https://doi.org/10.1177/10634266231154196

Lardier, D. T., Dickson, E. L., Hackett, J. M., & Verdezoto, C. S. (2023). A scoping review of existing research between 1990 and 2023: Measuring virtual communities of practice across disciplines. *Journal of Community Psychology, 52*, 198–225. https://doi.org/10.1002/jcop.23092

Lyon, A., Whitaker, K., Locke, J., Cook, C. R., King, K., Duong, M., Davis, C., Weist, M. D., Ehrhart, M., & Aarons, G. A. (2018). The impact of inter-organizational alignment (IOA) on implementation outcomes: Evaluating unique and shared organizational influences on education sector mental health. *Implementation Science, 13*, 24.

Mellin, E. A., & Weist, M. D. (2011). Exploring school mental health collaboration in an urban community: A social capital perspective. *School Mental Health, 3*(2), 81–92. https://doi.org/10.1007/s12310-011-9049-6

National Center for School Mental Health. (2023). *School mental health policy map.* School Health Assessment and Performance Evaluation (SHAPE) System, University of Maryland School of Medicine. https://theshapesystem.com/#policy-map

Newton, S., Horner, R., Algozzine, B., Todd, A., & Algozzine, K. M. (2009). Using a problem-solving model for data-based decision making in schools. In W. Sailor, G. Dunlap, G. Sugai, & R. Horner (Eds.), *Handbook of positive behavior support* (pp. 551–580). Springer.

Olivier, D. F., & Huffman, J. B. (2016). Professional learning community process in the United States: Conceptualization of the process and district support for schools. *Asia Pacific Journal of Education, 36*(2), 301–317. https://doi.org/10.1080/02188791.2016.1148856

Panchal, N., Cox, C., & Rudowitz, R. (2022, September 6). *The landscape of school-based mental health services.* KFF. https://www.kff.org/mental-health/issue-brief/the-landscape-of-school-based-mental-health-services/

Polanyi, M. (1962). *Personal knowledge: Towards a post-critical philosophy.* Chicago, IL: The University of Chicago Press.

Project ECHO. (n.d.). *University of New Mexico Health Sciences.* https://projectecho.unm.edu/

Pyrko, I., Dörfler, V., & Eden, C. (2017). Thinking together: What makes communities of practice work? *Human Relations, 70*(4), 389–409. https://doi.org/10.1177/0018726716661040

Pyrko, I., Dörfler, V., & Eden, C. (2019). Communities of practice in landscapes of practice. *Management Learning, 50*(4), 482–499. https://doi.org/10.1177/1350507619860854

Roberts, J. (2006). Limits to communities of practice. *Journal of Management Studies, 43*(3), 623–639.

Scaccia, J. P., Cook, B. S., Lamont, A., Wandersman, A., Castellow, J., Katz, J., & Beidas, R. S. (2015). A pradtical implementation science heuristic for organizational readiness: R = MC^2. *Journal of Community Psychology, 43*(4), 484–501. https://doi.org/10.1002/jcop.21698

Seguin, C. M., Culver, D. M., & Kraft, E. (2023). Knowledge translation and the untapped resource: Exploring the value of a community of practice for mental performance consultants. *Professional Psychology: Research and Practice, 54*(5), 342–351. https://psycnet.apa.org/doi/10.1037/pro0000514

Splett, J. W., Trainor, K., Raborn, A., Halliday-Boykins, C., Garzona, M., Dongo, M., & Weist, M. D. (2018). Comparison of universal mental health screening and traditional school identification methods for multi-tiered intervention planning. *Behavioral Disorders, 43*(3), 344–356.

Splett, J. W., Perales, K., Miller, E., Hartley, S., Wandersman, A., Halliday, C., & Weist, M. D. (2022). Using readiness to understand implementation challenges in school mental health research. *Journal of Community Psychology, 50*(7), 3101–3121.

Splett, J. W., Perales, K., Pohlman, K., Alquiza, K., Collins, D., Gomez, N., Houston-Dial, R., Meyer, B., & Weist, M. D. (2024). *Enhancing team functioning in schools' multi-tiered systems of support.* Center for Positive Behavioral Interventions and Supports (funded by the Office of Special Education Programs, U.S. Department of Education). Eugene, Oregon: University of Oregon Press. Retrieved from http://www.pbis.org

Struminger, B., Arora, S., Zalud-Cerrato, S., Lowance, D., & Ellerbrock, T. (2017). Building virtual communities of practice for health. *The Lancet, 390*(10095), 632–634. https://doi.org/10.1016/S0140-6736(17)31666-5

Waxman, R. P., Weist, M. D., & Benson, D. M. (1999). Toward collaboration in the growing education – Mental health interface. *Clinical Psychology Review, 19*, 239–253.

Wenger, E. (1998). *Communities of practice: Learning, meaning, and identity.* Cambridge University Press.

Wenger-Trayner, E., & Wenger-Trayner, B. (2015). *An introduction to communities of practice: A brief overview of the concept and its uses.* Available from authors at https://www.wenger-trayner.com/introduction-to-communities-of-practice

Wenger-Trayner, E., Wenger-Trayner, B., Reid, P., & Bruderlein, C. (2022). *Communities of practice within and across organizations: A guidebook.* Social Learning Lab.

Weist, M. D., Figas, K., Stern, K., Terry, J., Scherder, E., Collins, D., Davis, T., & Stevens, R. (2022). Advancing school behavioral health at multiple levels of scale. *Pediatric Clinics of North America, 69*(4), 725–737. https://doi.org/10.1016/j.pcl.2022.04.004

Wood, B. J., & McDaniel, T. (2022). A preliminary investigation of universal mental health screening practices in schools. *Children and Youth Services Review, 112*, 104943. https://doi.org/10.1016/j.childyouth.2020.104943

Chapter 4
School-Community Resource Mapping: A Foundational Practice for the Development of Effective School Mental Health Systems

Katherine A. Perkins, Kristen Figas, Darien Collins, and Elaine Miller

4.1 Introduction to Resource Mapping for Infrastructure Development

Mental health difficulties among children and youth have been increasing in prevalence over the past two decades (Centers for Disease Control and Prevention [CDC], 2019; Perou et al., 2013). Students spend seven hours per day on average in school; therefore, these difficulties are likely to present themselves and be exacerbated or improved by the school environment. With the best systems, programs, training, and supports in place, professionals can deliver high quality educational experiences while caring for children and themselves. Unfortunately, many school settings find themselves overwhelmed by challenges, inundated with potential solutions, and sometimes without a high level of control or agency. School-community resource mapping is a promising school or district-led practice for optimizing mental health support, including the integration of mental health programming and services with other mental health promoting resources.

Resource mapping (sometimes called asset mapping or environmental scanning) is a core practice in strategic infrastructure development. Developed as a strengths-based approach, resource mapping is community initiated and carried out for the

K. A. Perkins (✉)
Yvonne and Schuyler Moore Child Development Research Center,
University of South Carolina, Columbia, SC, USA
e-mail: kp40@mailbox.sc.edu

K. Figas · D. Collins
Department of Psychology, University of South Carolina, Columbia, SC, USA
e-mail: kfigas@email.sc.edu; darienc@email.sc.edu

E. Miller
University of Kansas, Lawrence, KS, USA
e-mail: elainemiller@ku.edu

purpose of locally directed development. Indeed, resource mapping has a prolific history in international and community development (Mathie & Cunningham, 2003; Mcknight, 2017; Peace Corps, 2007). It is often coupled with needs assessment and other strategic program and initiative planning practices. Whereas needs assessments are focused on deficits and problems, resource mapping offers the opportunity for communities to assess strengths and use those as a base for growth, regardless of the intensity of needs. For schools, school districts, and other local education agencies looking to grow their student supports and success, the application of resource mapping practice is an ideal starting point. In spite of this promise, little work has been done to assess the state of this practice in schools or the tools and methods employed.

In this chapter, we review freely available resource mapping tools, present and summarize their key features, and synthesize available literature on resource mapping practice in schools. We conclude with a discussion of systems thinking concepts in the context of resource mapping to guide the development or optimization of systems of support within schools with the intent of meeting the needs of every person. We emphasize that the presence of a formal multi-tiered system of support (MTSS) is not a prerequisite to resource mapping practice, but sustained efforts should logically lead to movement toward the development and strengthening of an MTSS (see Eber et al., 2020).

4.1.1 Identification of Available Tools

To identify resource mapping tools for review, we conducted three targeted Google searches in English. These searches returned 171 relevant results (116,000 total) for "school" AND "resource mapping," 191 relevant results (90,900 total) for "school" AND "asset mapping," and 198 relevant results (338,000 total) for "school" and "environmental scan." We excluded results identified as presentation materials and school- or district-specific maps, reports, and directories (products), resulting in 10 freely available resource mapping tools. We then searched the National Positive Behavior Interventions and Supports (PBIS) Technical Assistance website (www.pbis.org), a well-known resource repository for the more than 25,000 schools implementing PBIS, which did not populate any results in our three searches. We identified the "Technical Guide for Alignment" as a school resource mapping tool to be included in our in-depth review due to conceptual and content similarity, making a total of 11 technical resources intended for use by individuals or teams based in schools and/or school districts (local education agencies). Although our search was thorough, it was likely not exhaustive due to differences in terminologies used for this practice. Finally, we conducted a literature search for empirical papers presenting evidence on the use and effectiveness of resource mapping tools in school settings.

It is notable that the majority of search results were school and district products developed and made available online. Resources recovered through the "asset mapping" search were largely developed for community coalitions and organizations under the Asset-Based Community Development (ABCD) framework (Kretzmann et al., 2005). Search results under "environmental scan" tended to be school and district reports on both needs and resources at a point in time, rather than resource mapping tools. A number of non-profit, non-government organizations (NGO), academic, and government community development and education technical assistance organizations around the globe also came up in our search. Many offer services (some at no-cost) to facilitate and grow resource mapping practices in and out of school contexts but did not offer free technical tools online.

4.1.2 Essential Features of Resource Mapping Tools

Table 4.1 summarizes the essential features of the 11 resource mapping tools, organized chronologically by the date they were developed or last updated. This table can be used as a comparative reference for readers. Overall observations are summarized below from our detailed review of these products.

Audience

Although all tools were developed for use in schools or school districts (also referred to in resource mapping tools as local education agencies, including tribes or local territories), the audience varies in specificity and breadth. For instance, six tools are designed to be used by all school and/or district teams, whereas one is meant for high school teams serving students with autism. In addition, one tool is designed specifically for middle and/or high school teams, two are intended for use by leadership teams (e.g., social, emotional, behavioral, and mental health [SEBMH]) generally, and one is targeted specifically toward established MTSS teams. Resource mapping process materials include guidance for teaming under a variety of headings, including "pre-planning," "pre-mapping," "the alignment process," and sometimes "teaming."

Content Areas

All of the resource mapping tools cover a variety of topics, and each tool includes a unique combination of resource content areas for teams to consider. These are described in more detail in the "Resource Content Areas" column of Table 4.1. Four tools focus on mapping existing school resources, whereas seven of the tools take an explicitly integrative approach, guiding teams in mapping both school and community resources.

Table 4.1 Summary of resource mapping tool features

Tool	Audience	Resource content areas	Process	Tier Placement (MTSS)	Products for school or district	Products for service users	Community participation guidance
1. Iowa Safe Supportive Schools Grant (n.d.). *Iowa Safe Supportive Schools Continuum Mapping Guide.*	*All School and District Teams*	*School and Community Supports for Instruction* Community Partnerships Safe, Healthy, and Caring Learning Environments Child/Youth Engagement Support for Transition Parent Support and Involvement	*Partial Guidance and Worksheets* School Teaming Continuum Mapping Resource Mapping Evaluation	*Yes*	A continuum map with support organized by content area into "Core", "Supplemental", or "Intensive" A resource directory with suggested elements, including intervention framework, population served, personnel assigned, and funding allocations Analysis of gaps and duplication Product worksheet includes lines for indicating "Evidence-Based" and "Effectiveness Measured"	*Yes* Continuum map may be shared with students and families	Recommended but no guidance on roles or how this can be done

| 2. American Institutes for Research Safe Schools/Healthy Students Initiative SS/HS Framework Implementation Toolkit. (2012). *Conducting a Needs Assessment and Environmental Scan for a Safe Schools/Healthy Students Initiative in Your School and Community.* | District or School Leaders and Staff | School and Community Existing Resources, Services, and Systems (funding streams, policies, procedures, technology resources) | *Guidance and Worksheet* Needs Assessment Environmental Scan Gap Analysis (also addresses overlap, duplication, and coordination) Comprehensive Plan Building Partnerships *Links* to resources for implementing, sustaining, and expanding | No | List of needs by subpopulation, risk or protective factors, and indicators and data sources used List of existing Resources, Services, and Systems at the district/LEA/territory/tribe level (funding streams, policies, procedures, technology resources) Gap analysis framed as questions to consider | *No* None explicit | Community partnerships identified as the crux of all; partnership guidance brief and general "Four Simple Questions" developed by the IDEA (Individuals with Disabilities Act) to guide discussions |

(continued)

Table 4.1 (continued)

Tool	Audience	Resource content areas	Process	Tier Placement (MTSS)	Products for school or district	Products for service users	Community participation guidance
3. The Center on Secondary Education for Students with Autism (2012). *Community and School Resource Mapping.*	*High School Teams Serving Students with Autism Spectrum Disorders*	*School and Community Community:* Recreation and Religious Resources Employment Resources Vocational, Adult, and Continuing Education Independent Living and Transportation *School:* Case Manager Extracurricular Class Activities Community Service Technology Health Suite	*Guidance and Worksheets* Task Analysis Pre-Mapping (Teaming, Goals, Reflection) Mapping Post-Mapping (Communicate findings, review, update, evaluate)	*N/A* (For supporting students with autism)	List or directory of information by category for school teams, students, and families	*Yes* Organize information for student and family Create a visual structure for student	Recommended; little guidance on this beyond web searches and suggested community member roles on teams

4 School-Community Resource Mapping

3. Student Assistance Program Guidebook: A Resource for Schools developed by The Student Assistance Center at Prevention First. (2012). *Student Assistance Program Resource Map.*	*All School and District Teams*	*School and Community* Strength Based Resources Emotional Resources Social Resources Study Skills Resources Health Resources Academic Resources Behavioral Resources Other Resources	*Guidance* Program planning Placement of services and programs in tiers Alignment Family involvement Service coordination School/Community partnerships Sustainment *Links* to resources and tools Resource Map *Worksheet*	Yes	Master list of local resources that hold potential for developing partnerships or offer resources, assessment or treatment services for youth and families	*Yes* Student Assistance Program Services list for students, families, and community partners	General guidance
4. Lever et al. (2014). *Resource mapping in schools and school districts: A resource guide.*	*All School and District Teams* (and guidance for which)	*School and Community* All available resources/ programs for children, youth, and families in the school and surrounding community	*Guidance and Worksheets* Pre-mapping (e.g., purpose, teaming, history) Mapping Maintaining, Sustaining, and Evaluating	Yes	List of resources and Directory (with recommended data elements) Analysis: gaps, duplications, match with needs, underutilizations, outreach plan Outcome measures/ Evaluation	*Yes* Resource Information Sheet	Site visits recommended, student and family feedback recommended; little guidance on this involvement

(continued)

Table 4.1 (continued)

Tool	Audience	Resource content areas	Process	Tier Placement (MTSS)	Products for school or district	Products for service users	Community participation guidance
5. Center for Mental Health in Schools at UCLA. (Revised 2015). *Resource Mapping and Management to Address Barriers to Learning: An Intervention for Systemic Change.*	*All School and District Teams*	*School and Community* Programs Services Real estate Equipment Money Social capital Leadership Infrastructure mechanisms	*Guidance* and *Worksheets* Planning Teaming Mapping Resource Staff Mapping Programs, Activities, and Services Mapping funding and related resources (equipment, facilities) Mapping Community Resources Collating Policies Analyses	*No*	Reports by content area of resources and identified needs from students, teachers, and families Initial mapping list of products with program/service, grade level, eligibility, how to access, and number served List of coordinating professionals across schools	*Yes* Posters Social Marketing	Conceptual Framing and *Worksheets* for Inventorying and Selecting Community Outreach Efforts

6. Massachusetts Department of Elementary Education, Novak Educational Consulting, & Rodriguez Educational Consulting Agency (2017). *MTSS tiered resource map.*	*All School and District MTSS Teams*	*School Only* Curriculum and Instruction Assessments Data-based Decisions Divided into academic and social emotional/ Behavioral, and Mental Health Suggests districts may add other wellness domains	*Worksheets by TIER*	*Yes*	Comprehensive list of school's resources in chosen categories	*No* None Explicit	*None*
7. National Technical Assistance Center on Positive Behavior Interventions and Support (2017). *Technical Guide for Alignment of Initiatives, Programs and Practices in School Districts.*	*School District Leaders and Teams*	*School Only* Grants Initiatives Practices	*Guidance and Worksheets* Alignment self-assessment Alignment worksheet Identify and analyze MTSS core features Action planning for alignment References out to *Hexagon Tool* for evaluating fit and feasibility of new initiatives, programs, and services (Metz, A. & Louison, L., 2018)	*Yes*	A list of all grants, initiatives, and practices across schools and community agencies with indication of population served for valued outcomes and MTSS core system features (used to implement) Systems alignment action plan	*No* None Explicit	*None*

(continued)

Table 4.1 (continued)

Tool	Audience	Resource content areas	Process	Tier Placement (MTSS)	Products for school or district	Products for service users	Community participation guidance
8. Making Caring Common Project of the Harvard Graduate School of Education (2018, October). *Resource Mapping Strategy.*	*Middle School and High School Teams*	*School Only* Mental or Behavioral Health Supports Climate Building Activities or Initiatives Social Emotional Learning and Character Education	*Guidance and Woksheets* Pre-Planning Mapping Resources Analyzing Resources Maintaining Map Considering Changing Resources	*No*	Analysis: Gaps, redundancies, dependencies, rates of use, evaluation planning List of programs by type List of program details worksheet	*No* None explicit	*None*
9. National Center for School Mental Health, University of Maryland School of Medicine (2020). *School mental health quality guide: Needs assessment & resource mapping.*	*All School Teams*	*School and Community* List of suggestions, including Mental health services Housing Food Healthcare Mentoring After school programming Recreation	*Conceptual Guidance, Best Practices, and Links To Resources and Worksheets* Needs Assessment Resource Mapping Updating Resource Mapping Analysis and Decision-Making	*Yes*	Needs Assessment Report Comprehensive list of mental health resources and services Gap analysis, strategic alignment and abandonment	*Yes* User-friendly guide about mental health resources and services (suggested data elements listed)	Recommended; little guidance beyond roles

10. Education Development Center and Transforming Education for the MA Department of Elementary and Secondary Education (2021, March). *Social and Emotional Learning and Mental Health: Tiered Supports Inventory.*	*All School and District Teams*	*School Only* SEL and mental health programs, practices, and policies for students and families	*Guidance and Worksheets* Team Brainstorm Chart Resources Analyze for comprehensiveness	*Yes*	List of school—based programs by tier, populations served, lead or contact person, and implementation status Implementation Status Ratings: Suggest 3 levels of staff, student, and family buy-in alongside levels of staff training	*No* None Explicit	*None*

Mapping Process

Each tool offers a somewhat different approach to the resource mapping process. Most of the tools (10) provide explicit guidance on how to conduct resource mapping, which is helpful for school-based teams or leaders that may be new to the process. A number of the tools offer guidance on the different stages of the mapping process, such as planning/pre-mapping, mapping, maintenance/sustainment, and evaluation. Others, such as the *Student Assistance Program Resource Map* from the Student Assistance Center at Prevention First (2012), offer specific guidance on how to partner with communities and involve families. The resource mapping tool from the Center for Mental Health in Schools at UCLA (2015) provides detailed guidance on how to map specific types of resources, such as staff resources, activities/services, funding and logistical resources, and community resources. The amount of detail in the guidance varies by resource. All of the tools provide worksheets that teams can use to structure the resource mapping process and organize information they obtain, and three of the resource mapping tools also provide links to supplemental resources and tools.

Tier Placement

While only one of the resource mapping tools was designed expressly for "MTSS teams," seven of the tools offer tier placement options to help teams organize their resources into three tiers based on the resource's intended reach (see Table 4.1). A resource for all would fall into Tier 1, a resource provided to some would fall into Tier 2, and the most time or money-intensive resources would fall into Tier 3 for use with the fewest, as indicated. By prompting teams to consider the intensity of resources and the type of student needs they are most appropriate for, these tools can be helpful in easing resource navigation and decision making even if a school or district does not currently have a formal MTSS framework in place.

Products

All of the resource mapping tools include products that schools and districts can use to document resources and actions, but the products themselves vary. Some examples include resource directories with a variety of categorization schemes, detailed action plans, lists of partners, and data analysis approaches (e.g., to identify gaps, redundancies). A few of the resource mapping tools offer unique features. For instance, the National Center on School Mental Health *School Mental Health Quality Guide* (2020) includes a needs assessment report to help teams link needs assessment with resource mapping. The *Tiered Supports Inventory* from the Massachusetts Department of Elementary and Secondary Education (2017) includes products that focus on assessing buy-in, training and technical assistance needs, and dissemination planning to prompt teams to consider important process variables and plan for next steps.

In addition to providing useful products for schools and districts, six of the resource mapping tools provide user-friendly products for service users themselves (e.g., children, families, and staff). These products range from guidance and worksheets on tailoring and disseminating products to materials ready to be shared with children and families. Examples of these materials include maps and other visual resources, service lists and information sheets, posters and social marketing materials, and a user-friendly guide on mental health resources.

Community Participation Guidance

While the importance of partnerships is implicit in all of the resource mapping tools, only some of the tools speak to how to partner effectively with communities to collect information on community resources. Six of the tools provide brief guidance or simply recommend partnering with communities without offering any specific guidance. Four of the tools do not address this issue at all; however, one tool, from the Center for Mental Health in Schools at UCLA (2015), provides more substantial guidance, including worksheets for approaching and organizing community partnership efforts.

Time Commitment

Only three of the reviewed resource mapping tools suggest the time it will take to complete resource mapping. The Making Caring Common Resource Mapping Strategy (2018) suggests the process will take 30 minutes for mapping and 30 minutes to 1 hour for analysis. In *Resource Mapping and Management to Address Barriers to Learning: An Intervention for Systemic Change from the Center for Mental Health in Schools* (Center for Mental Health in Schools at UCLA, 2015), it is suggested to begin with a brief mapping before growing the practice to more in-depth procedures over the course of months. The American Institutes for Research Safe Schools/Healthy Students Initiative SS/HS Framework Implementation Toolkit (2012) suggests needs assessment and resource mapping should take place over the course of five months and comprehensive mapping over the course of seven months.

Evidence Base

There was a paucity of empirical literature on the practice of resource mapping, asset mapping, or environmental scanning in school settings. It is unknown how widespread the practice is, the characteristics and use of products generated by schools or districts that engage in this practice worldwide, or the effectiveness of resource mapping practice for systems building. There are a number of case studies and strong rationale for the practice (Crane & Mooney, 2005), as well promising program evaluation evidence from school counseling practice for serving specific populations locally (Arriero & Griffin, 2018; Griffin & Farris, 2010).

4.2 Synthesis and Discussion

The 11 reviewed resource mapping tools directed toward schools and school districts have considerable variability in character and content. Our reasonably large number of Google search hits resulting in presentations and local products indicates that this practice is somewhat popular among researchers, schools, and districts, primarily in the United States, and predominantly within the past 20 years.

It should be noted that some of the tools group mental health, social emotional learning, and behavior together within a single resource category. While these categories certainly overlap, they are not synonymous, and teams should be careful not to conflate them when examining resources. Grouping these categories together presents a risk of overlooking important elements. For example, an abundance of resources supporting student behavior may mask gaps in social emotional learning or mental health programs and services. Similarly, some may mistakenly conclude that delivering a social emotional learning curriculum is sufficient for meeting students' mental health needs. It is important that teams regard these conceptually related categories as offering distinct resources to ensure that the full spectrum of resources is mapped. When considering a resource mapping tool and deciding which resource elements to map, using a greater number and diversity of resource types can guard against approaching systems building too narrowly or too abstractly (Trochim et al., 2006). In addition, the amount and types of guidance across tools varies, so teams should be intentional in selecting a tool that provides adequate support.

Relatedly, a majority of resource mapping tools reviewed suggest placing programs and service resources into tiers. For those implementing a multi-tiered system of support (MTSS), this is likely intuitive. For those just starting out, the tier system indicates the intensity of a support, from Tier 1 universal supports (delivered to all student and/or staff), to Tier 2 supports (stronger intensity or modified support delivered to some), to Tier 3 supports (high intensity or individualized support given to few when indicated; see Eber et al., 2020). In order to have a multi-tiered system, schools must develop systems and policies for identification and referral (such as universal screening), service delivery (who and how), and progress monitoring (how to know something is helping and when we should change or stop). We recommend that schools at this stage of systems building development map their systems resources as well. Some tools, such as the Technical Guide for Alignment of Initiatives, Programs and Practices in School Districts (National Technical Assistance Center on PBIS, 2017), offer a template for mapping some of these systems.

There is a gap in the evaluation of evidence associated with programs and services in the majority of these mapping tools. Two templates give explicit space to document evidence. Many mention analyzing use and buy-in, but these factors can be closely tied to the quality of evidence and its presentation to the community. Schools and teams who would like explicit guidance on the evaluation of the evidence base for programs and services can visit resources given by the American Institutes for Research Safe Schools/Healthy Students Initiative SS/HS Framework Implementation Toolkit (2012) or National Center for School Mental Health, University of Maryland School of Medicine School Mental Health Quality Guide: Needs Assessment & Resource Mapping Tool (2020).

The extent to which a tool walks users through participatory analytic strategies beyond the production of lists/directories may give a more realistic picture of the effort involved and the possibilities for impact. Given that community participation guidance is somewhat limited, we recommend that leaders and teams looking for more structured support explore a community resource mapping tool such as Powerful Partnerships (Texas Workforce Commission Youth Program Initiative, 2003) and Participatory Asset Mapping: A Community Research Lab Toolkit (Burns et al., 2012). If teams are at a stage for mapping community partnerships, we suggest they consider distinguishing current and potential partnerships and keeping a detailed history of the partnership challenges and successes.

The National Center on Secondary Education and Transition Essential Tools: Community Resource Mapping (Crane & Mooney, 2005) is not reviewed above because it was identified as a community resource mapping tool, but in our screening of this tool, we noted that it explicitly suggests mapping resources at the state level. For this approach, pre-mapping involves the creation of a "task force" rather than a team that may deploy statewide surveys and host local community meetings across a state. It provides guidance and worksheets on building and sustaining partnerships as well as tailoring and disseminating products. Consensus building is the method for selecting mapping parameters. Resources created by law for a target population are governed by state and federal requirements, and systems building at this level for most schools and districts is typically through participation in state-level initiatives and advocacy efforts.

Finally, limited information on the time required suggests time investment can vary quite a lot based on the goals of the teams. Time studies would be a helpful avenue for researchers working to understand the balance of costs and benefits for resource mapping practice.

4.3   From Resource Mapping to Holistic Child, Youth, and Staff Well-Being

Children, youth, families, and schools exist in complex, sometimes volatile conditions. Historical, relational, cultural, political, and material forces shape and sustain each. Leaders in the fields of education, psychology, biology, public health, and sociology have offered discipline-defining theoretical models for how these forces interact to produce a vast number of outcomes (e.g., Bronfenbrenner, 1992; Von Foerster, 1952; Von Bertalanffy, 1972). In order for mental health support in schools to scale and sustain, we must shift from individual, organizational, and institutional capacity building to systems building, because the challenges we face transcend disciplines and isolated institutions.

A system is a set of interconnected elements that work together to perform a function or pursue a common purpose. Although a review of systems theories is beyond the scope of this chapter, there are a number of accessible resources on systems thinking for school leaders (e.g., Hayes, 2018; Shaked & Schechter, 2013). Half of the school-based resource mapping tools reviewed in this chapter treat resource mapping more as an inventory rather than an exploration or expansion process, although many do present systems building guidance encompassing resource integration or synthesis. With these strengths in mind, we next describe how seven major systems-thinking concepts can enhance school-community resource mapping research and practice going forward. Whether a school or district has formally adopted or fully implemented an MTSS framework or not, systems thinking during resource mapping practice can lay the groundwork for building optimally effective and efficient systems of student support.

4.3.1   Systems Thinking Concepts for Resource Mapping Research and Practice

Interconnectedness

We often fail to recognize that human development, needs, and behavior are complex and transcend isolated environments if we treat our resources, programs, and systems as independent and isolated parts. Disparate systems, programs, and services fulfilling interdependent needs can collectively surpass or suppress expected functioning depending upon our recognition of interconnectedness and subsequent systems building activities. Recognizing interconnectedness begins with humans, and the relationships between people are arguably the most critically important element for effective systems building. When well facilitated, interdisciplinary team members conducting resource mapping activities together can enhance one another's knowledge of systems, conceptual frameworks, service user experiences, and best practice through authentic relationship building. Consider a mental health training, where researchers found that school nurses expressed a need for mental health resource and referral training and the desire to grow skills in connecting with school teams (Bohnenkamp et al., 2019). It is not a stretch to imagine that many teachers and other school personnel would express some overlapping needs.

Systems mapping or building (when needed) is a logical part of resource mapping. This is particularly salient in professional development systems that incorporate or embed cross-professional programs and services in the educational setting. Overall, we recommend that (1) technical and professional development staff should be involved in developing any new partnership, program, or service adoption and (2) existing technical and professional development systems should be mapped as resources. When evaluating an initiative, consider if ongoing support can be made available and if there is a cost. The growth of government investment in national and state technical assistance centers in the United States, and the growth of coaching and consultation positions within education and human service systems means there are likely low- or no-cost options for major cross-system evidence-based programs, practices, and frameworks.

Many professional development systems in United States public schools operate in a top-down, insular fashion with little community involvement. Indeed, the majority of resource mapping tools we found have little concrete guidance on community involvement in resource mapping, even when it was highly recommended. A core purpose of this chapter is to demonstrate the value of an expanded or ground-up approach to the identification, adoption, and/or integration of the most helpful community and mental health resources for building and optimizing effective school-based systems of support. When selecting individuals for teams conducting resource mapping activities, it is helpful to choose people who have been formally trained in resource mapping facilitation or other participatory analytic methods. This likely includes individuals fulfilling roles mentioned in the resource mapping tools reviewed for this chapter, such as school administrators, counselors, psychologists, social workers, and teachers. Many teacher training programs, particularly those preparing individuals for alternate routes to licensure, include community asset mapping as a pedagogical practice, often with the explicit purpose of multicultural education, building relationships with students, and understanding roles within larger systems (Beck et al., 2022; Wheatley, 2006). Local universities, institutes of higher education, and community coalitions, such as United Way partnerships, can be a helpful no-cost source for resource mapping technical support.

Synthesis and Emergence

Emergence can be thought of as the overall functioning of integrated programs, practices, and systems that leads to the observable outcomes and impacts (e.g., mental health, physical health, and academics). Although many resource mapping tools suggest conducting a gap analysis between needs and resources and identifying redundancies and dependencies, there is no one way or right way to synthesize, align, and assess fit of programs, practices, and systems for integration. The Hexagon

Tool (Metz & Louison, 2018) offers a participatory consensus framework and guide for leaders and teams to choose implementation efforts. This tool is most suited for use in schools and districts that have already identified at least one potential new resource. Because of the time commitment, teams may aim to identify and evaluate a few options at once. On a basic level, researchers, leaders, and teams should evaluate ethical and methodological quality, consistency, and thoroughness in the integration of programs, practices, and systems (e.g., partnership, outreach, professional development, and funding). Emergent social behavior (also referred to in systems science as social self-organization) is an explanatory factor for systems-building outcomes and a promising avenue for future research on the effectiveness of resource mapping practice.

The synthesis of disparate programs, practices, and systems (e.g., education and mental health) often challenges our perceptions of what the problems are, what the solutions are, where professional boundaries should be drawn, and who the decision maker(s) should be. Moreover, partners discover they do not agree or perhaps do not agree right away. For example, during resource synthesis, practitioners in both educational and mental health service systems in the United States reported the same frequency and intensity of post-traumatic stress symptoms among the children, youth, and adults they work with, on average, but expressed differences in knowledge and access to training, the use of evidence-based practices, screening practices, and the availability of resources within their systems (Guevara et al., 2021). Guevara and colleagues also noted confusion among professionals when referring to trauma-informed evidence-based practices between school and community mental health practitioners (e.g. trauma-informed enhancements to PBIS curricula vs. Cognitive Behavioral Therapy frameworks), with a heavy emphasis on academic outcomes observed in some schools. Relationships (both connection and conflict) and data are foundational for integration and systems building.

Even if leaders or teams are only responsible for bringing to bear expertise in their own areas as is appropriate, holistic resource mapping conducted collectively and accessible to all may increase the likelihood that every caring adult in the building is up to date on the possible supports and the ways they are accessed and delivered in the school setting. With sustained practice, as new concerns arise, teams can check in with their systems mapping to see if a new resource is needed or if there are opportunities for functional improvement in the existing systems.

Pattern Recognition

Pattern recognition in the schooling context is one way to actively assess the emergent functioning of programs, practices, and subsystems as a whole and the extent to which they collectively deliver on the mission and vision of a school, district, or local education agency for every student. A wide range of data collection methodologies are suggested across resource mapping tools that can assist with systematic and targeted pattern recognition for student and family experiences and outcomes. These include questionnaires, surveys, interviews (both telephone and personal interviews), focus groups, roundtable discussions, written or oral public testimony, direct observation, consultation with people in key positions or with specific knowledge, review of relevant policies, review of public data (e.g., KIDS COUNT), and review of internal administrative data (discipline, attendance, grades). Disaggregating data by race, gender, ethnicity, language, disability, or other specified social group population can help schools assess how equitable and effective their system is and identify goals for improvement.

Feedback Loops

Feedback loops are an essential feature of well-functioning systems. In the context of resource mapping, two major feedback loops can be established through sustained practice: (1) the identification, mapping, and synthesis of new resources (either as an annual practice or in response to new evidence, relationships, or community resources) and (2) the identification of new concerns as described above in pattern recognition. Should a concern not be addressable through the existing system, a third feedback loop would be to trigger the purposeful identification, mapping, and synthesis of a matched resource. While the creation of resource directories may be fairly quick, the cultivation of new relationships and integration of new resources can take more time. The systems thinking concepts described so far are illustrated in Fig. 4.1.

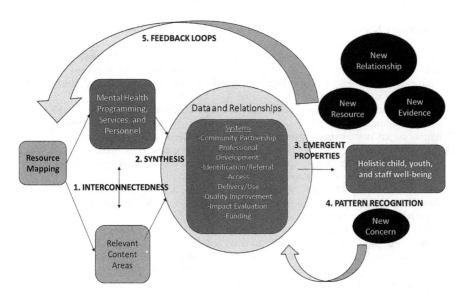

Fig. 4.1 Systems thinking for resource mapping research and practice

Causality and Systems Mapping

Lastly, in the process of resource mapping, many locales may find their options limited, particularly for the connection or integration of health and human services that meet their population needs. School leaders and teams can consider exploring causality (root causes) and systems mapping on a larger scale in this situation. Historical and ongoing racial and income segregation among schools in the United States, for example, have produced intergenerational school and district level disparities in resource access (Reardon & Owens, 2014; Owens et al., 2016). Researching and documenting the history of state and federal policy can offer insights and evidence for school community members to use when advocating for change in their own communities.

References

American Institutes for Research Safe Schools/Healthy Students Initiative SS/HS Framework Implementation Toolkit. (2012). *Conducting a needs assessment and environmental scan for a safe schools/healthy students initiative in your school and community.* Substance Abuse and Mental Health Services Administration. https://www.samhsa.gov/resource/ebp/safe-schoolshealthy-students-framework-implementation-toolkit

Arriero, E., & Griffin, D. (2018). ¡Adelante! A community asset mapping approach to increase college and career readiness for rural Latinx high school students. *Professional School Counseling, 22*(1), 2156759X18800279.

Beck, J. S., Lunsmann, C. J., & Moore, D. (2022). *Building community through asset mapping in an alternate route to licensure program.* The Professional Educator Advance Online Publication. https://digitalcommons.odu.edu/teachinglearning_fac_pubs/174

Bohnenkamp, J. H., Hoover, S. A., Connors, E. H., Wissow, L., Bobo, N., & Mazyck, D. (2019). The mental health training intervention for school nurses and other health providers in schools. *The Journal of School Nursing, 35*(6), 422–433.

Bronfenbrenner, U. (1992). *Ecological systems theory.* Jessica Kingsley Publishers.

Burns, J., Pudrzynska Paul, D., & Paz, S. (2012). *Participatory asset mapping: A community research lab toolkit.* https://communityscience.com/wp-content/uploads/2021/04/AssetMappingToolkit.pdf

Center for Mental Health in Schools at UCLA. (Revised 2015). *Resource mapping and management to address barriers to learning: An intervention for systemic change.* http://smhp.psych.ucla.edu/pdfdocs/resourcemapping/resourcemappingandmanagement.pdf

Centers for Disease Control and Prevention [CDC]. (2019). *Youth risk behavior survey: Data summary & trends report 2009–2019.* https://www.cdc.gov/healthyyouth/data/yrbs/pdf/YRBSDataSummaryTrendsReport2019-508.pdf

Crane, K., & Mooney, M. (2005). *Essential tools improving secondary education and transition for youth with disabilities: Community resource mapping.* https://dol.ny.gov/system/files/documents/2021/11/resource-resourcemapping-ncset.pdf

Eber, L., Barrett, S., Perales, K., Jeffrey-Pearsall, J., Pohlman, K., Putnam, R., Splett, J., & Weist, M. D. (2020). *Advancing education effectiveness: Interconnecting school mental health and school-wide PBIS, Volume 2: An implementation guide.* Center for Positive Behavioral Interventions and Supports (funded by the Office of Special Education Programs, U.S. Department of Education). Eugene, Oregon: University of Oregon Press. https://www.pbis.org/resource/interconnecting-school-mental-health-and-pbis-volume-2

Education Development Center and Transforming Education for the MA Department of Elementary and Secondary Education. (2021, March). *Social and emotional learning and mental health: Tiered supports inventory*. https://www.edc.org/sites/default/files/uploads/Tiered-Support-Inventory.pdf

Griffin, D., & Farris, A. (2010). School counselors and collaboration: Finding resources through community asset mapping. *Professional School Counseling, 13*(5), 2156759X1001300501.

Guevara, A. M. M., Johnson, S. L., Elam, K., Rivas, T., Berendzen, H., & Gal-Szabo, D. E. (2021). What does it mean to be trauma-informed? A multi-system perspective from practitioners serving the community. *Journal of Child and Family Studies, 30*(11), 2860–2876.

Hayes, F. (2018). Shaked, H., & Schechter, C. (2017). *Systems thinking for school leaders: Holistic leadership for excellence in education*. Springer.

Iowa Safe Supportive Schools Grant. (n.d.). *Iowa safe supportive schools continuum mapping guide*. National Center on Safe Supportive Learning Environments. https://safesupportive-learning.ed.gov/resources/iowa-safe-supportive-schools-continuum-mapping-guide

Kretzmann, J. P., McKnight, J., & Puntenney, D. (2005). *Discovering community power: A guide to mobilizing local assets and your organization's capacity*. Asset-Based Community Development Institute, School of Education and Social Policy, Northwestern University. https://wlcvs.org/wp-content/uploads/2015/07/ABCD_and_organisations.pdf

Lever, N., Castle, M., Cammack, N., Bohnenkamp, J., Stephan, S., Bernstein, L., Chang, P., Lee, P., & Sharma, R. (2014). *Resource mapping in schools and school districts: A resource guide*. Center for School Mental Health. https://dm0gz550769cd.cloudfront.net/shape/78/7836bc25375bed7ed2bc906407be674e.pdf

Making Caring Common Project of the Harvard Graduate School of Education. (2018, October). *Resource mapping strategy*. https://mcc.gse.harvard.edu/resources-for-educators/resource-mapping-strategy

Massachusetts Department of Elementary Education, Novak Educational Consulting, & Rodriguez Educational Consulting Agency. (2017). *MTSS tiered resource map*. Massachusetts Tools for Schools. https://matoolsforschools.com/resources/mtsstieredresourcemap

Mathie, A., & Cunningham, G. (2003). From clients to citizens: Asset-based community development as a strategy for community-driven development. *Development in Practice, 13*(5), 474–486.

McKnight, J. (2017). *Asset-based community development: The essentials*. Asset-Based Community Development Institute.

Metz, A., & Louison, L. (2018). *The hexagon tool: Exploring context*. National Implementation Research Network, Frank Porter Graham Child Development Institute, University of North Carolina at Chapel Hill. Based on Kiser, Zabel, Zachik, & Smith (2007) and Blase, Kiser & van Dyke (2013).

National Center for School Mental Health, University of Maryland School of Medicine. (2020). *School mental health quality guide: Needs assessment & resource mapping*. https://www.schoolmentalhealth.org/media/SOM/Microsites/NCSMH/Documents/Quality-Guides/Needs-Assessment-&-Resource-Mapping-2.3.20.pdf

National Technical Assistance Center on Positive Behavior Interventions and Support. (2017). *Technical guide for alignment of initiatives, programs and practices in school districts*. Center on PBIS. https://www.pbis.org/resource/technical-guide-for-alignment-of-initiatives-programs-and-practices-in-school-districts

Owens, A., Reardon, S. F., & Jencks, C. (2016). Income segregation between schools and school districts. *American Educational Research Journal, 53*(4), 1159–1197.

Peace Corps. (2007). *Participatory analysis for community action (PACA) training manual*. Peace Corps Information Collection and Exchange Publication, (M0053). https://files.peacecorps.gov/multimedia/pdf/library/PACA-2007.pdf

Perou, R., Bitsko, R. H., Blumberg, S. J., Pastor, P., Ghandour, R. M., Gfroerer, J. C., Hedden, S. L., Crosby, A. E., Visser, S. N., Schieve, L. A., Parks, S. E., Hall, J. E., Brody, D., Simile, C. M., Thompson, W. W., Baio, J., Avenevoli, S., Kogan, M. D., & Huang, L. N. (2013). Mental health surveillance among children–United States, 2005–2011. *Morbidity and Mortality Weekly Report, 62*(2), 1–35.

Reardon, S. F., & Owens, A. (2014). 60 years after Brown: Trends and consequences of school segregation. *Annual Review of Sociology, 40*, 199–218.

Shaked, H., & Schechter, C. (2013). Seeing wholes: The concept of systems thinking and its implementation in school leadership. *International Review of Education, 59*(6), 771–791.

Student Assistance Program Guidebook: A Resource for Schools developed by The Student Assistance Center at Prevention First. (2012). *Student Assistance program resource map.* https://www.prevention.org/Resources/c54b613c-d9d7-456d-99d2-2521e531e003/StudentAssistanceProgramGuidebook.pdf

Texas Workforce Commission Youth Program Initiative. (2003). *Powerful partnerships.* http://static1.1.sqspcdn.com/static/f/1003781/13662130/1344879052770/partnership1203.pdf?token=vIgA9KhHBaGqyRVWmLCvkTAHEls%3D

The Center on Secondary Education for Students with Autism. (2012). *Community and school resource mapping.* Frank Porter Graham Child Development Institute. https://csesa.fpg.unc.edu/resources/community-and-school-resource-mapping

Trochim, W. M., Cabrera, D. A., Milstein, B., Gallagher, R. S., & Leischow, S. J. (2006). Practical challenges of systems thinking and modeling in public health. *American Journal of Public Health, 96*(3), 538–546.

Von Bertalanffy, L. (1972). *The history and status of general systems theory.* Wiley-Interscience.

Von Foerster, H. (1952). *Cybernetics; circular causal and feedback mechanisms in biological and social systems.* Josiah Macy, Jr. Foundation.

Wheatley, M. (2006). *Leadership and the new science: Discovering order in a chaotic world.* Berrett-Koehler.

Chapter 5
Systematic Screening in Tiered Systems to Support Student's Well-Being

Kathleen Lynne Lane, Katie Scarlett Lane Pelton, and Wendy Peia Oakes

5.1 Systematic Screening in Tiered Systems to Support Student's Well-Being

Regardless as to where the political pendulum swings in terms of educational funding priorities, approaches to reading instruction, views on how to facilitate school safety, or other current trends, most educators agree on the goals of providing positive, productive, equitable, and safe learning environments for all students (Lane et al., 2021a, b). Furthermore, many educators would agree prevention is key, and it is desirable to detect and respond to challenges as early as possible—at the first sign of concern when challenges are more amenable to intervention efforts (Kauffman, 1999; Walker et al., 2004).

We see this often in the medical field. Health practices prioritize preventing high blood pressure, diabetes, and cancer through effective, relatively low-effort practices such as adequate sleep, nutrition, and fitness routines (Kauffman, 1999; Walker, 2017). In addition, people engage in routine screenings such as vision, hearing, blood panels, and other procedures (e.g., mammograms, blood pressure tests, intake questionnaires asking about family history and sleep routines) to check for characteristics or indicators predictive of important outcomes. For example, blood sugar levels predict pre-diabetes conditions, higher prostate-specific antigen (PSA)

K. L. Lane (✉)
University of Kansas, Lawrence, KS, USA
e-mail: Kathleen.Lane@ku.edu

K. S. L. Pelton
University of Connecticut, Storrs, CT, USA
e-mail: Katie.Lane@uconn.edu

W. P. Oakes
Arizona State University, Tempe, AZ, USA
e-mail: Wendy.Oakes@asu.edu

© The Author(s), under exclusive license to Springer Nature Switzerland AG 2024   81
L. Kern et al. (eds.), *Scaling Effective School Mental Health Interventions and Practices*,
https://doi.org/10.1007/978-3-031-68168-4_5

levels predict prostate cancer, and limited sleep predicts a host of negative outcomes (e.g., cognitive decline, heart disease, and diabetes; Walker, 2017). In these examples, screening is the first step to detecting potentially major diseases at the first indication of concern and—with the use of data sources (e.g., diagnostic tests)—informing intervention efforts.

The same is true in the field of education. Screening plays a key role in informing prevention efforts within the school context. For example, over the last several decades, reading screenings have been routine in many schools—particularly elementary schools—across the United States (Briesch et al., 2022). In optimal conditions, teachers conduct systematic screenings for reading and math performance in fall, winter, and spring each year using validated tools (e.g., aimswebPLUS, Pearson Assessment, 2016; DIBELS, University of Oregon, 2018–2019). This information is used to inform Tier 1 (see Chap. 2, this volume for a description of tiered support) reading and mathematics instruction for the school as a whole. Educators also use these data to guide instructional decisions for grade levels, specific classrooms, and individual students who might—despite the best possible instructional programming using validated strategies, practices, and programs—need more than Tier 1 practices have to offer. Before conducting any screenings, meticulous plans are detailed to design a coordinated continuum of support. Such plans feature adopting and installing validated resources to provide Tier 1 reading (e.g., 90 min daily English and language arts) and math (e.g., 60 min daily) instruction for all students, validated Tier 2 and Tier 3 interventions for students needing additional instruction, and guidance for data-inform decision making efforts.

Screening is also used to identify students' behavioral, social, and emotional well-being needs. Researchers and practitioners have partnered to study and refine systematic screening tools for use in PK -12th grade to support students' outcomes (Lane et al., 2024). In the 1990s, Hill Walker and others wisely prioritized detecting both major challenges of childhood and youth—externalizing (e.g., aggressive, non-compliant) and internalizing behaviors (e.g., socially withdrawn, anxious)—with the Systematic Screening for Behavioral Disorders (SSBD; Walker & Severson, 1992) initially designed for use at the elementary level and later expanded for use preschool through high school (Feil et al., 1995; Walker et al., 2015). The SSBD and other feasible screening tools (e.g., Student Risk Screening Scale; Drummond, 1994) provided the foundation for subsequent inquiry into screening not only from teacher perspectives, but also family and student perspectives.

During the last 30 years, the scope of available tools expanded dramatically, including strength-based screening tools, tools with versions that gather multiple perspectives, and tools with corresponding intervention materials (Kettler et al., 2014; Pelton et al., 2024). Some examples include the Behavior Assessment System for Children (third ed.); Behavioral and Emotional Screening System (BASC-3 BESS; Kamphaus & Reynolds, 2015); Devereux Student Strengths Assessment-mini (DESSA-mini; Naglieri et al., 2011, 2014); the Social, Academic, and Emotional Behavior Risk Screener© (SAEBRS; Kilgus et al., 2013); the Social Skills Improvement System–Performance Screening Guide or Social Emotional Learning (SSiS-PSG or SEL; Elliott & Gresham, 2008, 2015); the Strengths and

Difficulties Questionnaire (SDQ; Goodman, 2001); the Student Risk Screening Scale (SRSS; Drummond, 1994); the Early Identification System (EIS; Herman, et al., 2023); and the Student Risk Screening Scale–Internalizing and Externalizing (SRSS-IE; Drummond, 1994; Lane & Menzies, 2009).

The gift of early inquiry into teacher-completed screening tools was the ability to detect accurately both externalizing and internalizing behaviors with very limited teacher time (e.g., 15–30 min of total teacher time to screen an entire class; Oakes et al., 2017). This was—and remains—an important finding given the covert nature of internalizing behaviors (Walker et al., 2004) and well-established evidence documenting how the presence of externalizing and/or internalizing behaviors predicts a host of negative outcomes for students. Fall SRSS-IE screening scores can predict the number of office discipline referrals (ODRs) and days suspended over an academic year, as well as the number of visits to the nurse, number of course failures, and end of the year reading and math performance (Gregory et al., 2021; Lane et al., 2012, 2019a, b). Most recently, predictive validity studies demonstrated fall SRSS-IE screening scores even predicted referrals to special education (Lane et al., 2024).

Decades of studies have established many students with emotional and behavioral challenges (e.g., externalizing and/or internalizing behaviors) struggle with academic engagement and work completion, develop limited self-determined behaviors (e.g., decision-making, self-regulation), and experience school failure and ultimately school dropout (Nelson et al., 2004; Walker et al., 1996). Similarly, strained relationships with peers and authority figures during school continue into adulthood, manifesting in higher rates of accessing mental health supports, unemployment, underemployment, and divorce (Zablocki & Krezmien, 2013). These well-documented, short- and long-term negative outcomes suggest students do not "outgrow" externalizing and internalizing behaviors without intervention (Forness et al., 2012). Left unchecked, externalizing and internalizing behaviors give way to a range of challenges that impede students' well-being.

As such, it is imperative that educators prioritize systematic screening for early detection of behavior and well-being concerns. Similar to academic screening data, behavior screening data should be used along-side other sources of data (e.g., attendance, office discipline referrals, and nurse visits) for a comprehensive picture of students' progress to inform instruction for all students and connect those needing more than Tier 1 efforts to validated Tier 2 and Tier 3 interventions (e.g., counselor-led social skills instructions at Tier 2, school psychologist-led cognitive restructuring lessons). Additionally, these data can inform teacher practices and professional learning to help build their repertoire to maximize student engagement and establish a sense of belonging in classrooms (e.g., increased opportunities to respond; Common et al., 2020). This coordinated system of data-informed care (see Chap. 2, this volume) is needed to meet students' academic, behavioral, and social and emotional well-being learning needs (Behavior Analyst Certification Board, 2017; Office of the Surgeon General, 2021).

Since the late 1990s, the fields of education and school psychology have shifted to more integrated approaches to meeting students' multiple needs in school settings (McIntosh & Goodman, 2016). For example, we have seen broadening of traditional Response to Intervention (RTI, Fuchs & Fuchs, 2006) and Positive Behavior Intervention and Support (PBIS, Sugai & Horner, 2002) models now addressing multiple learning domains: Multi-Tiered System of Support (MTSS; McIntosh & Goodman, 2016), Integrated System Framework (ISF; Barrett et al., 2017), and Comprehensive, Integrated, Three-Tiered (Ci3T) models of prevention (Lane et al., 2009a, 2020a). With various nuances, these integrated tiered systems address students' academic, behavioral, and social and emotional well-being learning featuring a coordinated, data-information approach to instruction and professional learning (Briesch et al., 2022; Gandhi et al., 2020; Lane et al., 2020a).

Yet, screening tools for behavioral and social and emotional well-being are not as widely adopted as academic screening (Dineen et al., 2022; Bruhn et al., 2014). However, through the investments of the Institute for Education Sciences, educational leaders are prioritizing a systems level approach for meeting students' needs, with an increased emphasis on comprehensive, integrated tiered systems featuring systematic screenings—particularly teacher-completed screenings—conducted as part of regular school practices to meet students' multiple needs.

5.1.1 Purpose

In this chapter, we provide guidance for bringing systematic behavioral screening to scale within tiered systems to facilitate students' social and emotional well-being, featuring the Comprehensive, Integrated, Three-tiered (Ci3T) model of prevention as one type of integrated tiered system. As described in the introduction, systematic screening is a critical feature of all tiered systems to prevent the development of learning, behavioral, and social and emotional well-being challenges, as well as respond effectively when challenges arise. We offer three considerations for moving forward with systematic screenings in PK-12 school settings to support student's well-being. First, we recommend educational leaders establish clearly articulated, transparent plans for intervening at each level of prevention before introducing systematic screening tools and procedures. Second, we provide guidance for selecting an instrument that produces reliable scores, is valid for the school's intended use (e.g., informing instruction within tiered systems), and is practical tool for the school's context. Third, we address logistical considerations for installing the tool selected, including providing guidance for implementation practices. Throughout the chapter, we emphasize the role of professional learning for educators and community members to understand the value—and practicalities—of systematic screening to support students' well-being. We conclude with a summary as well as a listing of resources to support screening implementation and additional learning.

5.2 Establish a Plan for Intervening, *Before* Screening

First and foremost, it is important to have a plan for intervening before introducing systematic screening. In districts and schools implementing Ci3T, each school develops a Ci3T Implementation Manual to organize all the happenings at a school. Using a manualized professional learning process, school-site teachers work with district leaders to build Ci3T Implementation Manual using the following blueprints: (a) Primary (Tier 1) Plan, (b) Reactive Plan, (c) Expectation Matrix, (d) Assessment Schedule, (e) Secondary (Tier 2) Intervention Grid, and (f) Tertiary (Tier 3) Intervention Grid (Lane, Oakes, Cantwell et al., 2019; see ci3t.org/building for description the manualized Ci3T professional learning series). During our nearly three decades of collaborating with educators across the United States, we have learned there are many excellent strategies, practices, and programs in place in schools. Yet, in few cases are these elements organized into a comprehensive, transparent document available for all community members (e.g., faculty and staff, students, families, and administrators) to access. One example that accomplishes this goal is the Comprehensive, Integrated, Three-Tiered (Ci3T) model of prevention, which utilizes a written plan and the Ci3T Implementation Manual that delineates the integrated resources available to all students across academic, behavioral, and social and emotional well-being domains (Lane, 2017). More specifically, Ci3T is an integrated system, addressing district and state standards for academic instruction, Positive Behavioral Interventions and Supports (PBIS; Sugai & Horner, 2002) for the behavioral domain, and social and emotional well-being using validated resources. Ci3T can be viewed as a broadening of traditional Multi-Tiered System of Supports (MTSS; McIntosh & Goodman, 2016), which historically did not address social and emotional well-being. In addition to the Ci3T model of prevention facilitating data-informed instruction for students, it features data-informed professional learning for adults (Lane et al., 2020a).

For schools building their Ci3T model of prevention, there is a fully manualized professional learning process (Lane 2017) featuring a six-part series (3 full days and alternating three 2-hr sessions) spanning a single academic year. The full scope of professional learning materials is available at no cost on www.ci3t.org/build. Each school's Ci3T model is designed by a school-site Ci3T Leadership Team which includes the principal, two general education teachers, one special education teacher, another one or two professionals (e.g., counselor, school psychologist, interventionist), a family member, and the family member's child (who attends two of the 2-hr sessions; Lane et al., 2020a). In brief, the Ci3T Leadership Teams participate in a building process to develop a Ci3T model with the full-scope of evidence-based strategies, practices, and programs at each level of prevention: Tier 1 (for all), Tier 2 (for some), and Tier 3 (for a few). As part of this manualized building process, Ci3T Leadership Teams engage in a series of planned conversations and complete a set of Ci3T blueprints that result in a complete Ci3T Implementation Manual using the blueprint materials described above, with input from the full faculty and staff using a data-informed, iterative building process.

Within the Ci3T Implementation Manual, the Primary (Tier 1) Plan provides the mission and purpose, along with specific roles and responsibility for students, families, faculty and staff, and administrators for the academic, behavioral, and social and emotional well-being learning domains to ensure everyone in the school community knows how to contribute to student success. Furthermore, the plan includes procedures for teaching the components across these domains in an integrated fashion as well as procedures for reinforcing all contributing members (faculty and staff, students, and families). Given the importance of data-informed decision making in tiered systems, Tier 1 practices also detail step-by-step procedures for monitoring implementation in the fall and spring of each year. This ensures Tier 1 procedures for teaching, reinforcing, and monitoring are consistently implemented throughout the school by all those involved (Buckman et al., 2021; Lane et al., 2014). In addition, procedures for monitoring incorporated into the Ci3T Implementation Manual include guidance for conducting systematic screenings in fall, winter, and spring each year, and an assessment schedule (blueprint D) is included for adults to know when data from all sources are collected and available for decision making (Lane et al., 2020a). The Ci3T Implementation Manual provides educators with the framework to organize all available resources so they can swiftly connect students with appropriate supports once a need is detected.

To support implementation efforts, Ci3T Leadership Teams at each school continue their own professional learning, participating in a Ci3T Implementation Series, with five sessions during the academic year and one session during the summer, to review implementation and student performance data. Each session involves analyzing data to determine the professional learning needs for adults to inform their data-informed instruction for students. For example, during each year of Ci3T implementation, Ci3T Leadership Teams collaborate with district leaders to learn how to use screening data along with other data collected as part of regular school practices to (a) inform Tier 1 prevention efforts; (b) inform educators' use of teacher-delivered, low-intensity supports (e.g., behavior specific praise, Perez et al., 2023; instructional choice, Lane et al., 2023b); and (c) connect students with Tier 2 and Tier 3 intervention (Lane et al., 2014; Ma et al., 2021). For example, Ci3T Leadership Teams review summary data for the school as a whole to examine shifts in student performance over time (see Fig. 5.1 Panel A for externalizing behavior and Panel B for internalizing behavior).

Second, Ci3T Leadership Team members have opportunities to review multiple sources of data (see Fig. 5.2) and plan to conduct professional learning with faculty and staff to teach them the techniques and practices team members have learned during these team-based professional learning sessions. For example, during a 1-hr professional learning community (PLC) meeting, Ci3T Leadership Team members might join grade or department-level PLCs to review their data. If a teacher's fifth grade class indicated more than 20% of the students were in the high-risk level for internalizing behaviors, they might collaborate with the school psychologist or counselor to select additional lessons from their Tier 1 curriculum to support student well-being (e.g., how to identify and manage anxious feelings) which they may co-teach. During these lessons, the teacher and counselor might invite students

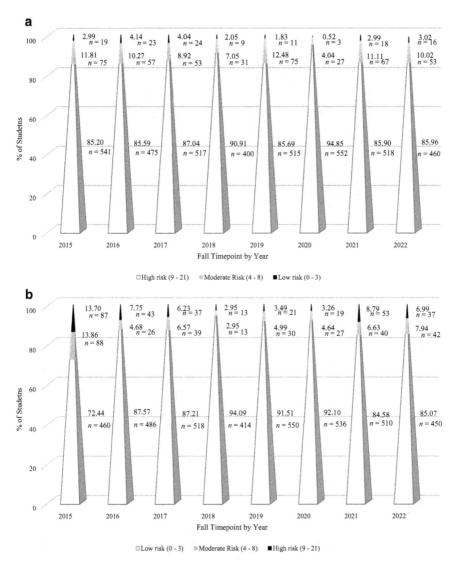

Fig. 5.1 Middle school fall screening scores over time. Panel A Fall SRSS-IE externalizing behaviors over time. Panel B Fall SRSS-IE internalizing behaviors over time. (Available on ci3t.org/PL)

experiencing moderate risk to participate in some of the modeling activities (e.g., role play scenarios) to glean further practice with those skills. Then, the teacher might pre-correct students on when to use these same strategies (e.g., positive self-talk) before engaging in activities that have proven stressful in the past for some students (e.g., group discussion, team-based sports during physical education).

Elementary Teacher Name: Wendy Peia
Date: September 19, 2023

Student Name	Student ID	AIMSweb Reading (1 Average or Above Average, 2 Below Average, 3 Well Below Average)	AIMSweb Math	Externalizing (0-3 Low, 4-8 Moderate, 9-21 High SRSS-IE)	Internalizing (0-3 Low, 4-8 Moderate, 9-21 High SRSS-IE)	ODR (0-1 Low, 2-5 Moderate, 6+ High)	Days Absent
Allen, Gale	123845	1	1	0	0	0	0
Brice, June	123846	2	1	4	9	3	0
Cambell, Mike	15248	1	2	0	0	0	1
Devon, Julius	123848	1	1	1	0	0	0
Dillaway, Marcus	94632	2	3	5	5	0	2
Evans, Tomas	123850	2	3	10	0	6	0
Flanagan, Ellen	257863	1	1	0	0	0	0
Garmin, Michaela	123852	3	1	1	10	0	2
Hankins, Kim	123853	1	1	0	0	0	0
Hu, Alec	257893	2	1	2	0	1	5
Illiad, Brian	257894	1	2	0	0	0	0
June, Scarlett	257895	1	1	0	8	0	1
Klien, Julio	254162	3	2	10	8	15	9
Lyon, Liam	257897	1	1	0	0	0	0
Montas, Craig	97851	1	2	0	5	0	0
Taylor, Elizabeth	99852	2	1	4	0	2	0
Willington, Helena	123861	1	3	0	5	0	3
Xan, Kathryn	258931	1	1	0	0	0	0

Fig. 5.2 Illustration of analyzing multiple sources of data at the elementary level

Secondary (Tier 2) Intervention Grid: For Middle and High School Students

Support	Description	School-Wide Data: Entry Criteria	Data to Monitor Progress	Exit Criteria
Self-monitoring	Strategy implemented by student and teacher to improve academic performance (completion/accuracy), academic behavior, or other target behavior	**Behavior** ☐ SRSS-E7 score: Moderate (4-8) *or* ☐ SRSS-E7 score: High (9-12) *or* ☐ 2 or more office discipline referrals (ODR) *or* ☐ Skyward: 2 or more course failures *or* ☐ Skyward: 2 or more missing assignments **AND/OR** **Academic** ☐ Report card: 1 or more course failures *or* ☐ AIMSweb: intensive or strategic level (math or reading) *or* ☐ Below 2.5 GPA	Work completion and accuracy of the academic area of concern (or target behavior named in the self-monitoring plan) Passing grades on progress reports **Social validity** Teacher: IRP-15 Student: CIRP **Treatment Integrity** Implementation & treatment integrity checklist	SRSS-E7 score: Low (1-3) Passing grade on progress report or report card in the academic area of concern (or target behavior named in the self-monitoring plan)

Fig. 5.3 Example of a secondary (Tier 2) intervention grid. (Available on ci3t.org/PL)

Third, Ci3T Leadership Teams learn how to implement interventions listed in the Secondary (Tier 2) and Tertiary (Tier 3) Intervention Grids (see Fig. 5.3 for an illustration of a Tier 2 intervention). These intervention grids feature the name of the intervention, a description (who is doing what to whom, and in what context; Horner et al., 2021), entry criteria (data reviewed to determine which students might need these extra supports), data reviewed during implementation (progress monitoring for students, along with treatment integrity, and social validity), and exit criteria (data reviewed to determine if they intervention should be faded, or if a more intensive intervention is needed). Ci3T Leadership Teams share what they learn from the Ci3T implementation series sessions with faculty and staff throughout the year as they move into implementation following the "building" academic year (see ci3t. org/imp for more information on the implementation series). For example, when creating the master calendar for each academic year, they schedule grade- or department-level meetings as well as district- and school-site professional learning offerings, indicating which data will be reviewed at each meeting. Ci3T Leadership Teams might share school-wide data summarized in aggregate form (see Fig. 5.1 for an illustration of how externalizing and internalizing data are summarized for the school as a whole) during the first 15 min of a professional learning session, followed by a work block for grade- or department-level teams to review their respective data to determine which students might need Tier 2 or 3. Educators can contact families and students to explore the most appropriate intervention from those listed in their Ci3T Implementation Manuals. It is important for families and students (depending on developmental stage and age) to be involved in the planning process about which intervention might be best suited to support engagement and well-being. For example, if a student shares a self-monitoring intervention form on their desk would be embarrassing, then a subtler procedure (e.g., placing the form on the inside front cover of a notebook) or use of technology might be preferred or perhaps a different intervention altogether (check/in, check/out, or direct behavior ratings).

As illustrated, it is important to have a systematic plan for intervening in place before screening begins. If screenings also included parent- or student-completed measures in addition to teacher-completed tools, it is imperative these data are reviewed quickly and accurately to determine if there are any immediate needs (e.g., if the student is in danger, or a danger to themselves and others; Lane et al., 2021a). Thanks to the investments of the Institute of Education Sciences (IES; see Lane et al., 2021b) and the Office of Special Education Programs (OSEP; Sherod et al., 2020), there are now volumes written on how to select, install, and interpret screening data (Oakes et al., 2018)—including how to communicate with the local community (Sherod et al., 2020). In the subsequent sections, we provide guidance for moving forward with systematic screening efforts, beginning with considerations for selecting a screening tool with attention to issues of reliability, validity, *and* practicalities.

5.3   Select a Screening Tool: Reliable Scores, Valid Inferences, and Practical for Your Context

Educational leaders preparing to implement universal behavior screening are faced with an important, though challenging, decision—selecting a screening tool. Typically, this decision takes place at the district level with input from school-site principals and an established leadership team (e.g., school-site Ci3T Leadership Team). A recent scoping review of studies evaluating universal behavior screening instruments identified over 50 instruments for detecting behavior patterns character- istic of emotional and behavioral problems in preschool through 12th grade students (Pelton et al., 2024). The plethora of available instruments presents an opportunity for educational leaders to find an instrument which has been thoroughly studied in a context similar to their own school. We present a framework for comprehensively evaluating potential instruments for adoption, including both practical consider- ations and psychometric properties.

With so many available instruments, we recommend starting by considering the age group of the students you are serving. Many screeners are developed for specific age groups (i.e., early childhood, elementary, secondary), so educational leaders can immediately limit their search to instruments normed for their age group of interest (Oakes et al., 2022). Most universal behavior screening research has been conducted within elementary schools, followed by middle schools and high schools, with the least in early childhood settings (Pelton et al., 2024). Given the limited research base in secondary and early childhood settings, this first step may substantially narrow the search for an instrument in those settings. Often districts prefer to install one screening tool for use elementary through high school levels, which narrows the selections as well.

Second, we recommend leaders determine their construct, in this case a specific behavior pattern, of interest (Oakes et al., 2017). Emotional and behavioral problems contain a wide range of behaviors, though they are primarily categorized into internalizing and externalizing behaviors (Walker et al., 2015). Different screening instruments may focus on different behaviors characteristic of emotional and behavioral problems or take different approaches such as strengths-based screening (e.g., motivation to learn; prosocial behavior; see Table 1 in Pelton et al., 2024). Although related, these different constructs are not necessarily interchangeable (Lane et al., 2023a). We encourage educational leaders to carefully consider their intended use of behavior screening scores to help focus on their construct of interest. For example, is the goal to detect internalizing behaviors as well as externalizing behaviors? or is the goal to assess self-regulation or prosocial behaviors?

Validity refers to the extent that an instrument measures what it is intended to measure. Therefore, it is important to remember the constructs measured by each tool's scores must align with the intended use to allow for strong evidence of a valid decision (Kane, 2013). For example, if your school or district is looking for students who are struggling with internalizing behaviors such as anxious feelings, withdrawal from social interactions with their peers, or somatic complaints, then it is important to make certain the tool selected is designed to detect internalizing behaviors. To clarify, no single instrument can be valid for all possible uses, so it is up to educational leaders to select an instrument which closely aligns with their intended use in practice.

By the third step, the instrument pool should be narrowed down enough to begin looking into each tool more closely. To ensure long-term feasibility, we recommend leaders consider the resources necessary to implement and maintain these screening instruments for many years to come as scores from screening tools are easy to compare for those interested in monitoring shifts in risk over time (Oakes et al., 2022). Cost is a key consideration for a sustainable system (Oakes et al., 2017). Cost includes the price of purchasing the screening instrument, professional learning for key personnel to use the system, and setting up the screening platform. Additionally, teachers need time to complete the screening process, so a lengthy screener could be costly during implementation. In most cases, commercially available screening instruments, such as the BASC-3 BESS or SiSS-PSG, may require less preparation time, though free-access screeners may be more feasible in the long term with only internal costs to implement. As such, no single instrument will be the best option for

Table 5.1 Resources to support systematic screening to facilitate student well-being

Resource	Location
American Education Research Association, American Psychological Association, and National Council of Measurement in Education (2014)	American Education Research Association: https://www.aera.net/ Publications/Books/ Standards-for-Educational-Psychological-Testing-2014-Edition
Center of PBIS: Positive Behavioral Supports and Interventions. (2019). *Systematic Screening Tools: Universal Behavior Screeners.* Center on PBIS, University of Oregon. www.pbis.org	Center of PBIS: Positive Behavioral Supports and Interventions https://www.pbis.org/resource/ systematic-screening-tools-universal-behavior-screeners
Comprehensive, Integrated, Three-Tiered (Ci3T) Model of Prevention. *Systematic Screening.* Author	https://www.ci3t.org/screening
Comprehensive, Integrated, Three-Tiered (Ci3T) Model of Prevention. *Systematic Screening: Setting Up to Screening in Your District or School.* Author	https://www.ci3t.org/screening Student Risk Screening Scale Internalizing and Externalizing
Comprehensive, Integrated, Three-Tiered (Ci3T) Model of Prevention. *Systematic Screening: Site Level Preparation Protocol.* Author	https://www.ci3t.org/screening Student Risk Screening Scale Internalizing and Externalizing
Systematic screening for behavior in current K-12 Settings. Lane et al. (2020b)	Center of PBIS: Positive Behavioral Supports and Interventions https://www.pbis.org/resource/ systematic-screening-for-behavior-in-current-k-12-instructional-settings
Universal screening – systematic screening to shape instruction: Lessons learned & practicalities. Lane et al. (2020c)	Center of PBIS: Positive Behavioral Supports and Interventions https://www.pbis.org/resource/ universal-screening-systematic-screening-to-shape-instruction
Interpreting universal behavior screening data: Questions to consider. Ma et al. (2021)	Center of PBIS: Positive Behavioral Supports and Interventions https://www.pbis.org/resource/ interpreting-universal-behavior-screening-data-questions-to-consider
Michigan Multi-tiered Assistance Center. *SRSS-IE Coordinator Resources.* Author. www.ci3t.org/ screening	https://www.ci3t.org/screening
Michigan Multi-tiered Assistance Center. *SRSS-IE Coordinator Training Resources.* Author. www.ci3t. org/screening	https://www.ci3t.org/screening
Selecting a universal behavior screening tool: Questions to consider. Oakes et al. (2021a)	Center of PBIS: Positive Behavioral Supports and Interventions https://www.pbis.org/resource/ selecting-a-universal-behavior-screening-tool-questions-to-consider

(continued)

Table 5.1 (continued)

Resource	Location
Guidance for systematic screening: Lessons learned from practitioners in the field. Oakes et al. (2021b)	Center of PBIS: Positive Behavioral Supports and Interventions https://www.pbis.org/resource/guidance-for-systematic-screening-lessons-learned-from-practitioners
Installing a universal behavior screening tool: Questions to consider. Oakes et al. (2022)	Center of PBIS: Positive Behavioral Supports and Interventions https://www.pbis.org/resource/installing-a-universal-behavior-screening-tool-questions-to-consider
Installing a universal behavior screening tool: Questions to consider. Schonour et al. (2022)	Center of PBIS: Positive Behavioral Supports and Interventions https://www.pbis.org/resource/the-whys-and-hows-of-screening-frequently-asked-questions-for-families
Screening coordinator training manual: a guide for installing the SRSS-IE in your school or district. Rollenhagen et al. (2021)	https://www.ci3t.org/screening > Student Risk Screening Scale Internalizing and Externalizing
Systematic screening in tiered systems: lessons learned at the elementary school level. Sherod et al. (2023)	Center of PBIS: Positive Behavioral Supports and Interventions https://www.pbis.org/resource/systematic-screening-in-tiered-systems-lessons-learned-at-the-elementary-school-level

all schools as many schools will have different resources available (see Table 5.1 for resources to guide decision-making efforts).

The final, and most time-consuming, step involves evaluating the psychometric properties of the instruments to determine whether they align with a given school's student population, construct of interest, and available resources. Psychometric studies on universal behavior screening date back to 1987 with a substantial increase in research published in the last 15 years (Pelton et al., 2024). The large body of literature on universal behavior screening demonstrates an ongoing commitment from researchers to ensure high-quality instruments are available for practitioners, though we recognize this may present practical challenges for educators. Here we provide a brief primer for psychometric evidence broadly organized into categories: reliability and validity.

Reliability is the proportion of true variation in scores out of the total variation in observed scores (McDonald, 1999). In theory, if each teacher could complete the same screener on the same students, in the same time frame many times, we would expect to observe highly similar results if the scores produced by the screener represent true variation in student behavior. Yet, if the instrument is highly susceptible to measurement error, we would likely see a high degree of variation in scores due to unknown factors other than student behavior. Of course, researchers cannot ask teachers to repeat the same measure several times for the same students in a very short period of time, so researchers estimate reliability with other methods. The most common reliability analysis with behavior screeners is a statistical estimate of internal consistency called coefficient alpha which estimates the degree to which items within a scale are related to one another (Cronbach, 1951; Pelton et al., 2024). Other methods include test-retest reliability, which involves asking the same person to complete the screening process twice for their students in a relatively short time frame to assess screening score stability (where the two scores are similar). Alternatively, some researchers study inter-rater reliability which involves two or more people completing the screener for the same student with the assumption highly similar ratings indicate accurate measurement of the student's behaviors, rather than the influence of other factors. In short, reliability is an estimate of the proportion of true variation due to student behavior out of all variation in scores; thus, high reliability is important for measuring true variation in student behavior.

As mentioned previously, *validity* relates to the inferences made using screening scores. The most common validity-related analyses for universal behavior screening are confirmatory factor analysis (CFA) and correlating screening scores to other theoretically related constructs (Pelton et al., 2024). CFA is a statistical procedure for seeing how well items form related groups as hypothesized by the researcher (Brown, 2006). Researchers often attribute a well-fitting CFA model to construct validity because it suggests observed item scores relate to a single, underlying construct (e.g., internalizing or externalizing or prosocial behavior)—the precise focus of construct validity (Shadish, et al., 2002). Other analyses examine how closely the score on the screener is similar to other theoretically related variables such as other screeners, behavior rating scales, or educational outcomes (e.g., attendance, office discipline referrals [ODRs], suspensions). The most common analysis for these studies is a correlation between two measures (Pelton et al., 2024). A correlation ranges from -1.0 to 1.0, indicating the direction and strength of the relationship between two observed scores (e.g., the relation between externalizing behaviors and number of ODRs; Taylor, 1990). Broadly, these comparison studies help researchers determine how well the instrument measures the construct of interest. For a more in-depth explanation of reliability and validity evidence, we refer readers to *The Standards for Educational and Psychological Testing* (American Education Research Association, American Psychological Association, & National Council for Measurement in Education, 2014). Also, we refer interested readers to supplemental Table 3 from Pelton et al. (2024) recent literature review which lists included studies by screening tool. For each article in this table, findings are summarized in an online supplemental file to help educators select a screening tool appropriate for the age-rage of students served, to look for the major constructs your school leaders are interested in, the reliability of the scores selected, and the validity of scores in predicting important outcomes for students.

Educational leaders are faced with a critical decision when selecting a screening instrument. With over 50 instruments available, there is sure to be a good fit, though it may be difficult to find. We recommend first determining the student population of interest and then the construct of interest to narrow down the list of potential instruments. From here, we recommend considering the resources needed to implement the screening tool initially and over time to ensure a sustainable system will be in place for years to come. Finally, we encourage leaders to thoroughly examine the psychometric evidence available for their final few options to determine which instrument produces reliable scores and has evidence of valid inferences aligned with their intended use. After educators select a validated tool, the next step is to develop implementation practices for the selected tools within the context of your schools' tiered system.

5.4   Develop Implementation Practices for Screening Tools Selected

With the important decision of selecting the screening tool that best fits with the goals and context of the school or school district, there are additional considerations and planning needed to establish strong implementation practices (Ma et al., 2021; Lane et al., 2020c; Oakes et al., 2014, 2022; Sherod et al., 2020). We recommend school leaders develop plans for preparing to screen, conducting each administration, ensuring accurate interpretation, and responding when screening scores indicate students may require Tier 2 or 3 interventions or supports.

5.4.1   Preparing

To prepare for screening, we recommend school leaders allocate financial and human resources to ensure screening practices and corresponding professional learning activities are adopted and sustained over time, including communicating with educators and families about the purpose of screening and how data will be used to promote student learning and other school outcomes. Advanced planning supports educators in efficiently and accurately completing screening for each student, accessing data for decision making, and feeling confident when talking with students' families about screening.

Over the past few years, with increased attention to meeting students' social and emotional well-being needs and the adoption of universal screening practices (Dineen et al., 2022; National Center for Educational Statistics, 2022; Office of the Surgeon General, 2021), there have been considerable investments in the development of online data management platforms that aid educators in collecting, managing, and using screening data. Companies offer secure platforms for collecting and managing screening data for school systems (e.g., Aperture Education, 2009; Illuminate Education, 2016; Pearson Assessments, 2016; Standard Co, 2023) with a range of management fees. Yet, limited financial resources do not preclude schools from successful implementation of screening. Schools may select a free-access measure such as the Student Risk Screening Scale for Internalizing and Externalizing behaviors (SRSS-IE; Drummond, 1994; Lane & Menzies, 2009). District data leaders then build the selected free-access screener into their existing data management system or create a secure way to collect and use screening data within secure shared drives. An important consideration is to ensure the data management system, whether purchased or built, is easy for educators to access compatible with other student-level data systems so that school leaders and educators may examine multiple sources of data for decision making (Kalberg et al., 2010). Further, we encourage leaders to ensure the systems selected are secure and meet local, state, and federal laws meeting Family Education Rights Act (FERPA) requirements for protecting sensitive student data.

Most often schools identify screening leaders at the school sites and at the district level (Oakes et al., 2022). At the district level, a screening coordinator takes responsibility for keeping site level screening leaders up to date with the three screening windows (fall, winter, and spring), and any shifts in the screening measures over years, and assures data are accessible for decision making by appropriate educators. District and school-site leaders organize professional learning for new and returning educators in the purpose, collection, and use of screening (see Rollenhagen et al. 2021). School-site screening leaders are often responsible for ensuring screeners are available during the screening window, leading meetings for teachers to come together to complete their individual screeners on the students in their assigned class period (for secondary) or homeroom (for elementary) to receive support, responding to any questions during screening, ensuring all students are screened during each window, and leading professional learning for accurate detection of students who may need additional supports and planning for appropriate responses (Oakes et al., 2021a, b). Often it is helpful to develop coaching protocols for school-site and district-level leaders to make these steps transparent and build institutional knowledge (see Table 5.1 links to sample coaching protocols).

Planned professional learning is recommended so that teachers feel confident in the purpose of screening, administration of the selected screening measure, and use of screening data for instructional decision making. School leaders can communicate with families about their behavior screening practices just as they do all other screening and assessment practices (Schonour et al., 2022). For example, schools may screen for hearing, vision, scoliosis, reading skills, or math skills. It is important for families to know when screening is occurring and how the information is used to inform Tier 1 instructional for all, empower teachers with low-intensity strategies, and assist their child if a Tier 2 or 3 intervention is needed. As noted above, we strongly encourage families and students to be involved in selecting and designing logistics for validated Tier 2 and 3 interventions. We encourage educators to consider how shared screening results may be interpreted by families and consider ways to teach families about this practice without adding undue concern (see Sherod et al., 2020). School leaders may consider having their family organization or school-site council review and offer feedback on any 'form' letters that may be used (e.g., notification of screening practices, information regarding opt out, communication of screening results). With a fully developed plan for initiating Tier 2 and 3 interventions in place as discussed in previous sections of this chapter, the structures for safely and accurately collecting screening data in place, and communication with the school community, screening is ready to begin as part of regular school practices for all students enrolled in a school.

5.4.2 Conducting

District and school-site screening leaders prepared to lead screening efforts including being fluent with the data collection system and fully understanding the developer's recommendations for completing the selected screening tool. We recommend school-site screening leaders create opportunities for teachers to come together to complete screening for each student, ensuring educators new to the district or school receive professional learning about the hows and whys of systematic screening during their onboarding activities and before screenings take place (see Oakes et al., 2014; Schonour et al., 2022). Benefits of this practice are that (a) giving teachers the time to complete the screeners shows respect for their time and that schools value of the importance of the data for supporting students, (b) screening leaders are available to clarify any misunderstandings about screening, and (c) screening leaders can support teachers in navigating the data collection platform and making sure all entered scores are saved (Oakes et al., 2022).

We offer a few considerations based on lessons learned with district partners over the past two decades (also see Oakes et al., 2021a, b). Ask teachers to check their prepopulated screening roster to ensure the correct class—particularly important at the secondary level—and the complete list of students are included. Students who have been enrolled for fewer than 30 days are typically not screened at a specific time point so that teachers have ample time to get to know the student and become familiar with their behavior patterns. In this case, students would be screened at the next scheduled time point. Technical guidance from the screener developer should provide directions on this point, if not, we recommend using the 30-day rule (e.g., Walker et al., 2015).

When conducting screening, the measures should be completed independently by the assigned teacher and not through group discussion and consensus. Unless otherwise noted in the technical guidance from the developers, screening tools are validated for use with independent teacher ratings. When teachers with assigned students are on long-term leave or have left their position, the screening leaders should ensure those students are screened by a teacher or other professional familiar with the students. The screening adult may be a long-term substitute (if there for at least 30 days), a related arts teacher, or a paraprofessional who works closely with the students, as a few possibilities. Professionals asked to screen in place of an unavailable teacher are provided the professional learning prior to screening so they can accurately complete the screeners. If teachers work on teams and share a roster of students (Basile et al., 2023), the missing teachers' students can be redistributed among the team members. The important point is that each student is screened to ensure (a) information is gleaned on the entire student body to examine Tier 1 practices and (b) early detection of concerns and the provision of appropriate interventions or supports.

5.4.3   Interpreting and Responding

With advancements in data management tools for screening (e.g., Illuminate Education, 2016) that are often compatible with other school data systems and increased availability of customization in existing platforms, scoring and interpretation have become efficient and accurate processes. For example, systems automatically score screeners so that teachers can see scores for individual students at the time of screening. Commercial platforms have reporting features for educators and school leadership teams to examine data for decision making at multiple levels. District leadership teams can look at risk levels by building, by grade, for groups with specific characteristics (e.g., students receiving special education), or make other comparisons guided by their improvement plans or priorities.

District leaders often consider resource allocation such as mental health providers, school counselors, or tiered interventions ensuring resources are mobilized and invested to support areas of identified need (see Chap. 4, this volume). Likewise, curricular and professional learning needs are examined. For example, data may show a school could benefit from instruction of Tier 1 social skills curriculum for all students or targeted groups of students at Tier 2 (Kilgus & Eklund, 2016). In the case of schools implementing Ci3T, decisions might be made to add additional lessons to the Tier 1 resources already implemented as part of regular school practices (e.g., bringing in additional lessons on self-regulation to manage anxious feelings if internalizing scores for the school as a whole suggest more than 20% of students are in the moderate or high risk level). District leaders and Ci3T Leadership teams examine screening alongside other student outcome data also considering treatment integrity (Tiered Fidelity Inventory [TFI], Algozzine et al., 2014) and social validity data (Lane et al., 2009b). Schools with lower levels of implementation of Tier 1 practices (i.e., treatment integrity) or social validity data, indicating educators may not agree with the goals or believe the procedures need refinement, will want to consider specific professional learning for faculty and staff to increase the use of Tier 1 practices so that students may benefit from their tiered system.

As discussed previously, school leadership teams (e.g., social, emotional, behavioral, and mental health [SEBMH]) are encouraged to review aggregated data for the school as a whole (Fig. 5.1) to examine the effectiveness of their Tier 1 practices, by grade level, by individual teacher, and by student (Ma et al., 2021). We recommend school (and district) level review always be considered alongside treatment integrity and social validity data. For tiered systems, such as Ci3T or PBIS, to have the intended impact on student outcomes, leaders must ensure they are implemented with fidelity before interpreting student outcomes (Buckman et al., 2021). Simply put, even the most effective system will not result in positive outcomes if not implemented as designed. Finally, teachers review their class data as a whole and by individual students (Fig. 5.2). If their data show more than 20% of their students are scoring in moderate- or high-risk ranges for behavior challenges or below academic benchmarks, teachers may first reflect on their individual implementation of their Tier 1 plan. For example, they may ask—are they using low intensity strategies such as behavior specific praise (Perez et al., 2023), precorrection (Sherod et al., 2023), instructional choice (Lane et al., 2023b), or increasing opportunities to respond (Common et al., 2020)? Are they teaching, offering opportunities to practice, and providing reinforcement for students to learn and use expected behaviors? Are they embedding social skill practice within academic lessons to allow students to engage in socially supportive ways (Lane et al., 2018)?

As illustrated, there are a number of important logistical considerations for installing the tool selected, including providing guidance for implementation practices. Just as it is important to establish a plan for intervening before introducing systematic screening efforts and select a psychometrically strong tool aligned with the school's goals, it is important to address the practicalities: preparing, conducting, as well as interpreting and responding.

5.5 Summary

In this chapter, we offered guidance for bringing systematic screening to scale within tiered systems to facilitate students' well-being. As described at the onset, systematic screening practices using reliable, valid, and practical tools are essential to achieve the goals of providing positive, productive, equitable, and safe learning environments from early childhood through the high school years. Information gleaned from screening tools can inform a range of learning opportunities for students and systems-level practices for the school as a whole to prevent academic, behavioral, and social and emotional well-being challenges from occurring. In addition, this information can be used to empower teachers with practical, effective low-intensity supports to maximize productive academic and social engagement in schools, as well as detect and respond to challenges at the first sign of concern when the discrepancy between current and desired performance patterns is most narrow (Kauffman, 1999; Walker et al., 2004).

Given systematic screening is a critical feature of all tiered systems, we detailed four considerations for educators committed to adopting systematic screenings in pre-K-12 school settings to support student's well-being. First, we encouraged educational leaders to develop transparent plans for intervening at each level of prevention (Tier 1 for all, Tier 2 for some, and Tier 3 for a few) before introducing systematic screening tools and procedures. It is important to have a plan for intervening before introducing systematic screening practices. Second, we provided guidance for selecting a tool which produces reliable scores, allows for valid inferences, and is practical for the specific context. It is important for educational leaders to know their state and local laws with respect to systematic screening, particularly when incorporating parent- and student-completed screening tools. Remember, teachers are mandated reporters. If they suspect a student is a danger to themselves or others, or if they are in harm's way, they are required to report this concern. Although we have focused primarily on teacher-completed screening tools in this chapter, it is important to note that when parent- and student-completed screenings are introduced, this brings in new information requiring immediate scoring, review, and response. Third, we address logistical considerations for installing the tool selected, including providing guidance for implementation practices. Specifically, we overviewed the practicalities of systematic screening: preparing, with attention to security and FERPA requirements; administration of the screening procedures with fidelity; interpreting; and responding. We illustrated the importance of professional learning for educators and community members to understand the value— and practicalities—of systematic screening to support well-being. It is important to develop professional learning plans to not only launch initial installation, but also continue screening practices with high fidelity (e.g., on boarding new teachers, examining data over time). We are hopeful the content of this chapter will be useful to educators—practitioners and researchers—committed to early detection across the preK-12 continuum. For the interested reader, we include other resources in Table 5.1 to facilitate screening to support well-being.

References

Algozzine, B., Barrett, S., Eber, L., George, H., Horner, R., Lewis, T., Putnam, B., Swain-Bradway, J., McIntosh, K., & Sugai, G. (2014). *School-wide PBIS tiered fidelity inventory.* OSEP Technical Assistance Center on Positive Behavioral Interventions and Supports. www.pbis.org

American Education Research Association, American Psychological Association, and National Council of Measurement in Education. (2014). *Standards for educational and psychological testing.* AERA. https://www.aera.net/Publications/Books/Standards-for-Educational-Psychological-Testing-2014-Edition

Aperture Education. (2009). *DESSA aperture system.* Author.

Barrett, S., Eber, L., & Weist, M. (2017). *Advancing educational effectiveness: Interconnecting school mental health and school-wide positive behavior support.* https://www.pbis.org/resource/advancing-education-effectiveness-interconnecting-school-mental-health-and-school-wide-positive-behavior-support

Basile, C. G., Maddin, B. W., & Audrain, R. L. (2023). *The next education workforce: How team-based staffing models can support equity and improve learning outcomes.* Rowman & Littlefield.

Behavior Analyst Certification Board. (2017). *BCBA task list* (5th ed.). Author.

Briesch, A., Lane, K. L., Common, E. A., Oakes, W. P., Buckman, M. M., Chafouleas, S. M., Sherod, R. L., Abdulkerim, N., & Royer, D. J. (2022). Exploring views and professional learning needs of Comprehensive, Integrated, Three-Tiered (Ci3T) leadership teams related to universal behavior screening implementation. *Education and Treatment of Children, 45,* 245–262. https://doi.org/10.1007/s43494-022-00080-8

Brown, T. A. (2006). Confirmatory factor analysis for applied research. .

Bruhn, A. L., Woods-Groves, S., & Huddle, S. (2014). A preliminary investigation of emotional and behavioral screening practices in K–12 schools. *Education and Treatment of Children, 37*(4), 611–634. https://doi.org/10.1353/etc.2014.0039

Buckman, M. M., Lane, K. L., Common, E. A., Royer, D. J., Oakes, W. P., Allen, G. E., Lane, K. S., & Brunsting, N. C. (2021). Treatment Integrity of primary (tier 1) prevention efforts in tiered systems: Mapping the literature. *Education and Treatment of Children, 44*(3), 145–168. https://doi.org/10.1007/s43494-021-00044-4

Common, E. A., Lane, K. L., Cantwell, E. D., Brunsting, N. C., Oakes, W. P., Germer, K. A., & Bross, L. A. (2020). Teacher-delivered strategies to increase students' opportunities to respond: A systematic methodological review. *Behavioral Disorders, 45*, 67–84. https://doi.org/10.1177/0198742919828310

Cronbach, L. J. (1951). Coefficient alpha and the internal structure of tests. *Psychometrika, 16*, 297–334. https://doi.org/10.1007/BF02310555

Dineen, J. N., Chafouleas, S. M., Briesch, A. M., McCoach, D. B., Newton, S. D., & Cintron, D. W. (2022). Exploring social, emotional, and behavioral screening approaches in U.S. public school districts. *American Educational Research Journal, 59*(1), 146–179. https://doi.org/10.3102/00028312211000043

Drummond, T. (1994). *The Student Risk Screening Scale (SRSS)*. Josephine County Mental Health Program.

Elliott, S. N., & Gresham, F. M. (2008). *Social skills improvement system: Performance screening guides*. Pearson Assessments.

Elliott, S. N., & Gresham, F. M. (2015). *Social Skills improvement system: Social and emotional learning*. Pearson Assessments.

Feil, E. G., Walker, H. M., & Severson, H. H. (1995). The Early Screening Project for young children with behavior problems. *Journal of Emotional and Behavioral Disorders, 3*(4), 194–202. https://doi.org/10.1177/106342669500300401

Forness, S., Freeman, S., Paperella, T., Kauffman, J., & Walker, H. (2012). Special education implications of point and cumulative prevalence for children with emotional and behavioral disorder. *Journal of Emotional and Behavioral Disorders, 20*(1), 4–18. https://doi.org/10.1177/1063426611401624

Fuchs, D., & Fuchs, L. (2006). Introduction to response to intervention: What, why, and how valid is it? *Reading Research Quarterly, 41*(1), 93–99. https://doi.org/10.1598/RRQ.41.1.4

Gandhi, A. G., Clemens, N., Coyne, M., Goodman, S., Lane, K. L., Lembke, E., & Simonsen, B. (2020). Integrated multi-tiered systems of support (I-MTSS): New directions for supporting students with or at risk for learning disabilities. In *Handbook of learning disabilities* (3rd ed.). Guildford Press.

Goodman, R. (2001). Psychometric properties of the Strengths and Difficulties Questionnaire (SDQ*). Journal of the American Academy of Child and Adolescent Psychiatry, 40*, 1337–1345. https://doi.org/10.1097/00004583-200111000-00015

Gregory, C., Graybill, E. C., Barger, B., Roach, A. T., & Lane, K. (2021). Predictive validity of the Student Risk Screening Scale-Internalizing and Externalizing (SRSS-IE) scores. *Journal of Emotional and Behavioral Disorders, 29*(2), 105–112. https://doi.org/10.1177/1063426620967283

Herman, K. C., Reinke, W. M., Thompson, A. M., Huang, F., & Owens, S. (2023). Usability and social consequences of the early identification system as a universal screener for social, emotional, and behavioral risks. *School Psychology, 38*(3), 148–159. https://doi.org/10.1037/spq0000538.supp

Horner, R., Blintz, C., & Ross, S. W. (2021). *The importance of contextual fit when implementing evidence-based interventions*. Office of the Assistant Secretary for Planning and Evaluation, U.S. Department of Health and Human Services. https://aspe.hhs.gov/reports/importance-contextual-fit-when-implementing-evidence-based-interventions

Illuminate Education. (2016). *Use social-emotional behavior assessments to support social-emotional learning*. Author. https://www.illuminateed.com/products/fastbridge/social-emotional-behavior-assessment/

Kalberg, J. R., Lane, K. L., & Menzies, H. M. (2010). Using systematic screening procedures to identify students who are nonresponsive to primary prevention efforts: Integrating academic and behavioral measures. *Education and Treatment of Children, 33*(4), 561–584. https://doi.org/10.1353/etc.2010.0007

Kamphaus, R. W., & Reynolds, C. R. (2015). *BASC-3 behavior and emotional screening system (BASC-2 BESS)*. Pearson.

Kane, M. T. (2013). Validating the interpretations and uses of test scores. *Journal of Educational Measurement, 50*(1), 1–73. https://doi.org/10.1111/jedm.12000

Kauffman, J. M. (1999). How we prevent the prevention of emotional and behavioral disorders. *Exceptional Children, 65*(4), 448–468. https://doi.org/10.1177/001440299906500402

Kettler, R. J., Glover, T. A., Albers, C. A., & Feeney-Kettler, K. A. (2014). *Universal screening in educational settings: Evidence-based decision making for schools*. American Psychological Association.

Kilgus, S. P., & Eklund, K. R. (2016). Consideration of base rates within universal screening for behavioral and emotional risk: A novel procedural framework. *School Psychology Forum Research in Practice, 10*(1), 120–130.

Kilgus, S. P., Chafouleas, S. M., Riley-Tillman, T. C., & von der Embse, N. P. (2013). *Social, academic, and emotional behavior risk screener: Teacher rating scale*. University of Missouri.

Lane, K. L. (2017). Building strong partnerships: Responsible inquiry to learn and grow together TECBD-CCBD keynote address. *Education and Treatment of Children, 40*, 597–617.

Lane, K. L., & Menzies, M. H. (2009). *Student risk screening scale for internalizing and externalizing behaviors* (SRSS-IE). Available at http://www.ci3t.org/screening

Lane, K. L., Kalberg, J. R., Bruhn, A. L., Driscoll, S. A., Wehby, J. H., & Elliott, S. N. (2009a). Assessing social validity of school-wide positive behavior support plans: Evidence for the reliability and structure of the Primary Intervention Rating Scale. *School Psychology Review, 38*(1), 135–144. https://doi.org/10.1080/02796015.2009.12087854

Lane, K. L., Kalberg, J. R., & Menzies, H. M. (2009b). *Developing schoolwide programs to prevent and manage problem behaviors: A step-by-step approach*. Guilford Press.

Lane, K. L., Menzies, H. M., Oakes, W. P., Lambert, W., Cox, M., & Hankins, K. (2012). A validation of the Student Risk Screening Scale for internalizing and externalizing behaviors: Patterns in rural and urban elementary schools. *Behavioral Disorders, 37*(4), 244–270. https://doi.org/10.1177/019874291203700405

Lane, K. L., Oakes, W. P., & Magill, L. (2014). Primary prevention efforts: How do we implement and monitor the tier 1 component of our comprehensive, integrated, three-tiered (ci3t) model? *Preventing School Failure: Alternative Education for Children and Youth, 58*(3), 143–158. https://doi.org/10.1080/1045988X.2014.893978

Lane, K. L., Oakes, W. P., Buckman, M. M., & Lane, K. S. (2018). *Supporting school success: Engaging lessons to meet students' multiple needs*. Council for Children with Behavior Disorders (CCBD) Newsletter.

Lane, K. L., Oakes, W. P., Cantwell, E. D., Common, E. A., Royer, D. J., Leko, M., Schatschneider, C., Menzies, H. M., Buckman, M. M., & Allen, G. E. (2019a). Predictive validity of Student Risk Screening Scale for Internalizing and Externalizing (SRSS-IE) scores in elementary schools. *Journal of Emotional and Behavioral Disorders, 27*(4), 221–234. https://doi.org/10.1177/1063426618795443

Lane, K. L., Oakes, W. P., Cantwell, E. D., & Royer, D. J. (2019b). *Building and installing Comprehensive, Integrated, Three-tiered (Ci3T) models of prevention: A practical guide to supporting school success* (v1.3). KOI Education.

Lane, K. L., Menzies, H. M., Oakes, W. P., & Kalberg, J. R. (2020a). *Developing a schoolwide framework to prevent and manage learning and behavior problems* (2nd ed.).

Lane, K. L., Oakes, W. P., Buckman, M. M., Sherod, R., & Lane, K. S. (2020b). *Systematic screening for behavior in current K-12 Settings*. Center on PBIS, University of Oregon. https://www.pbis.org/resource/systematic-screening-for-behavior-in-current-k-12-instructional-settings

Lane, K. L., Powers, L., Oakes, W. P., Buckman, M. M., Sherod, R., & Lane, K. S. (2020c). *Universal screening – Systematic screening to shape instruction: Lessons learned & practicalities*. Center on PBIS, University of Oregon. https://www.pbis.org/resource/universal-screening-systematic-screening-to-shape-instruction

Lane, K. L., Oakes, W. P., & Menzies, H. M. (2021a). Considerations for systematic screening PK-12: universal screening for internalizing and externalizing behaviors in the COVID-19 era. *Preventing School Failure: Alternative Education for Children and Youth, 65*(3), 275–281. https://doi.org/10.1080/1045988X.2021.1908216

Lane, K. L., Royer, D. J., & Oakes, W. P. (2021b). Literacy instruction for students with emotional and behavioral disorders: A developing knowledge base. In R. Boon, M. Burke, & L. Bowman-Perrot (Eds.), *Literacy instruction for students with emotional and behavioral disorders (EBD): Research-based interventions for the classroom* (pp. 1–17). Information Age Publishing.

Lane, K. L., Oakes, W. P., Monahan, K., Smith, A., Lane, K. S., Buckman, M. M., Lane, N. A., & Sherod, R. (2023a). A comparison of DESSA-mini and SRSS-IE screening tools. *Education and Treatment of Children., 46*, 367. https://doi.org/10.1007/s43494-023-00106-9

Lane, K. S., Buckman, M. M., Iovino, E. A., & Lane, K. L. (2023b). Incorporating choice: Empowering teachers and families to support students in varied learning contexts. *Preventing School Failure, 67*(2), 106–114. https://doi.org/10.1080/1045988x.2023.2181304

Lane, K. L., Oakes, W. P., Buckman, M. M., Lane, N. A., Lane, K. S., Fleming, K., Swinburne Romine, R., Sherod, R. L., Chang, C., & Cantwell, E. D. (2024). Additional evidence of predictive validity of SRSS-IE scores with elementary students. *Behavioral Disorders, 49*, 189. https://doi.org/10.1177/0198742923122289

Ma, Z., Sherod, R., Lane, K. L., Buckman, M. M., & Oakes, W. P. (2021). *Interpreting universal behavior screening data: Questions to consider*. Center on PBIS, University of Oregon. https://www.pbis.org/resource/interpreting-universal-behavior-screening-data-questions-to-consider

McDonald, R. P. (1999). *Test theory: A unified treatment*. Erlbaum.

McIntosh, K., & Goodman, S. (2016). *Integrating multi-tiered systems of support: Blending RTI and PBIS*. Guilford Press.

Naglieri, J. A., LeBuffe, P. A., & Shapiro, V. (2011). *Devereux student strengths assessment-mini*. Kaplan Press.

Naglieri, J. A., LeBuffe, P. A., & Shapiro, V. B. (2014). *The Devereux Student Strengths Assessment – mini (DESSA-mini): Assessment, technical manual, and user's guide*. Apperson.

National Center for Educational Statistics. (2022, July 6). *More than 80 percent of U.S. Public schools report pandemic has negatively impacted student behavior and socio-emotional development*. Institute of Education Sciences. https://nces.ed.gov/whatsnew/press_releases/07_06_2022.asp

Nelson, J. R., Benner, G. J., Lane, K., & Smith, B. W. (2004). Academic achievement of K-12 students with emotional and behavioral disorders. *Exceptional Children, 71*, 59–73. https://doi.org/10.1177/001440290407100104

Oakes, W. P., Lane, K. L., Cox, M., & Messenger, M. (2014). Logistics of behavior screenings: How and why do we conduct behavior screenings at our school? *Preventing School Failure, 58*, 183–190. https://doi.org/10.1080/1045988x.2014.895572

Oakes, W. P., Lane, K. L., Cantwell, E. D., & Royer, D. J. (2017). Systematic screening for behavior in K-12 settings as regular school practice: Practical considerations and recommendations. *Journal of Applied School Psychology, 33*, 369–393. https://doi.org/10.1080/1537790 3.2017.1345813

Oakes, W. P., Lane, K. L., Common, E. A., & Buckman, M. M. (2018). Systematic screening for behavior in early childhood settings: Early identification and intervention within a tiered prevention framework. *Perspectives on Early Childhood Psychology and Education, 3*, 10–38.

Oakes, W. P., Buckman, M. M., Lane, K. L., & Sherod, R. L. (2021a). *Selecting a universal behavior screening tool: Questions to consider*. Center on PBIS, University of Oregon. https://www.pbis.org/resource/selecting-a-universal-behavior-screening-tool-questions-to-consider

Oakes, W. P., Lane, K. L., Sherod, R. L., Adams, H. R., & Buckman, M. M. (2021b). *Guidance for systematic screening: Lessons learned from practitioners in the field*. Center on PBIS, University of Oregon. https://www.pbis.org/resource/guidance-for-systematic-screening-lessons-learned-from-practitioners

Oakes, W. P., Lane, K. L., Ma, Z., Sherod, R., & Pérez-Clark, P. (2022). *Installing a universal behavior screening tool: Questions to consider.* Center on PBIS, University of Oregon. https://www.pbis.org/resource/installing-a-universal-behavior-screening-tool-questions-to-consider

Office of the Surgeon General. (2021). *Protecting youth mental health: The U.S. Surgeon General's advisory.* https://www.hhs.gov/sites/default/files/surgeon-general-youth-mental-health-advisory.pdf

Pearson Assessments. (2016). *aimswebPLUS.* Author.

Pelton, K. S. L., Lane, K. L., Oakes, W. P., Buckman, M. M., Royer, D. J., & Sherod, R. L. (2024). *Mapping the research base for universal behavior screeners.* LDbase. https://doi.org/10.33009/ldbase.1711468821.4a16

Pérez, P., Gil, H., Artola, A., Royer, D. J., & Lane, K. L. (2023). Behavior-specific praise: empowering teachers and families to support students in varied learning contexts. *Preventing School Failure: Alternative Education for Children and Youth, 67*(2), 83–90. https://doi.org/10.1080/1045988X.2023.2181303

Rollenhagen, J., Buckman, M. M., Oakes, W. P., & Lane, K. L. (2021). *Screening coordinator training manual: A guide for installing the SRSS-IE in your school or district.* Author. https://www.ci3t.org/screening

Schonour, S. D., Lane, K. L., Oakes, W. P., Sherod, R. L., & Buckman, M. M. (2022). *The whys and hows of screening: Frequently asked questions for families.* Center on PBIS, University of Oregon. https://www.pbis.org/resource/the-whys-and-hows-of-screening-frequently-asked-questions-for-families

Shadish, W. R., Cook, T. D., & Campbell, D. T. (2002). *Experimental and Quasi-experimental designs for generalized causal inference.* Cengage Learning.

Sherod, R. L., Oakes, W. P., Lane, K. L., & Lane, K. S. (2020). *Tips for communicating with your community about systematic screening.* Center on PBIS, University of Oregon. https://www.pbis.org/resource/tips-for-communicating-with-your-community-about-systematic-screening-what-does-your-district-and-school-leadership-team-need-to-know

Sherod, R. L., Jones, J. S., Perry, H., & Oakes, W. P. (2023). Precorrection: empowering teachers and families to support students in varied learning contexts. *Preventing School Failure: Alternative Education for Children and Youth, 67*(2), 91–97. https://doi.org/10.1080/1045988X.2023.2181302

Standard Co. (2023). *Introduction to standard data – All of your district data in one place* [video]. Author. https://www.youtube.com/watch?v=ioJoS_gWYWU

Sugai, G., & Horner, R. (2002). The evolution of discipline practices: School-wide positive behavior supports. *Child & Family Behavior Therapy, 24*(1–2), 23–50. https://doi.org/10.1300/J019v24n01_03

Taylor, R. (1990). Interpretation of the correlation coefficient: A basic review. *Journal of Diagnostic Medical Sonography, 6*(1), 35–39. https://doi.org/10.1177/875647939000600106

University of Oregon. (2018–2019). *8th edition of dynamic indicators of basic early literacy skills (DIBELS®).* Author. https://dibels.uoregon.edu

Walker, M. (2017). *Why we sleep: Unlocking the power of sleep and dreams.* Simon & Schuster.

Walker, H. M., & Severson, H. (1992). *Systematic screening for behavior disorders: User's guide and technical manual.* Sopris West.

Walker, H. M., Horner, R. H., Sugai, G., Bullis, M., Spragues, J. R., Bricker, D., & Kaufman, M. J. (1996). Integrated approaches to preventing antisocial behavior patterns among school-age children and youth. *Journal of Emotional and Behavioral Disorders, 4*, 194–209.

Walker, H. M., Ramsey, E., & Gresham, F. M. (2004). *Antisocial behavior in school: Evidence-based practices* (2nd ed.). Wadsworth.

Walker, H. M., Severson, H., & Feil, E. G. (2015). *Systematic screening for behavior disorders* (2nd ed.). Ancora.

Zablocki, M., & Krezmien, M. P. (2013). Drop-out predictors among students with high-incidence disabilities: A National Longitudinal and Transitional Study 2 analysis. *Journal of Disability Policy Studies, 24*(1), 53–64. https://doi.org/10.1177/1044207311427726

Chapter 6
Just-in-Time Training

Samuel D. McQuillin, Amanda L. Davis, and Savannah B. Simpson

6.1 Introduction to Just-in-Time Training

In the late nineteenth century at the dawn of psychological science, the experimental psychologist Hermann Ebbinghaus discovered one of the first facts produced by a psychological experiment: people tend to forget things they learn (Ebbinghaus, 2013). He also found that this forgetting occurs at an exponential rate but can be curtailed by reviewing information. Though common sense to most, the simple act of reviewing information can be a matter of life or death in some circumstances. For example, when surgeons review and complete checklists prior to surgery, the rates of complications and subsequent deaths are reduced by 40–80% (Haynes et al., 2009). Similar observations are found in a range of industries, including aviation, heavy machinery operation, and construction, among others (Gawande, 2010). In these industries, much of routine professional practice, and subsequent success in reducing disaster, involves proactive efforts to reduce forgetting.

Although less ubiquitous than in industries where forgetting causes catastrophic events (e.g., aviation), forgetting also impacts the delivery of effective mental health services. For example, when clinicians attend training workshops in the counseling style Motivational Interviewing (MI), a particular counseling style that targets behavior change, these trainings produce strong effect sizes on MI knowledge, skills, and attitudes, yet most of these gains are lost within 2 months (Madson et al., 2009; Miller et al., 2004; Schwalbe et al., 2014; Smith et al., 2012). It is somewhat ironic that the positive effects of receiving MI as a client—which can be observed

S. D. McQuillin (✉) · S. B. Simpson
Department of Psychology, University of South Carolina, Columbia, SC, USA
e-mail: mcquills@mailbox.sc.edu; SBS16@email.sc.edu

A. L. Davis
Department of Psychology, Elon University, Elon, NC, USA
e-mail: adavis126@elon.edu

L. Kern et al. (eds.), *Scaling Effective School Mental Health Interventions and Practices*,
https://doi.org/10.1007/978-3-031-68168-4_6
105

nearly a year after treatment—can outlast the skills of their clinician by roughly 10 months. Similar results are found in a wide range of psychotherapy and intervention research, which has caught the attention of implementation scientists. A study by Sibley et al. (2021) found that implementation fidelity—the extent to which individuals implemented or used an intervention as it was intended to be used—for a randomized trial of a family-based attention-deficit/hyperactivity disorder (ADHD) treatment substantially declined across sessions of the multisession program, and these declines predicted worse outcomes for the families being served. In other words, implementation was strong when it was in close proximity to the training but declined dramatically as time went on, which is precisely what we would expect from Ebbinghaus's seminal studies. Thus, forgetting appears to be one factor that compromises how well mental health clinicians implement interventions and help people. Moreover, while forgetting learned skills or practices is a threat to performance, this assumes that learning occurred in the first place. However, in many circumstances, the threat to performance (or underperformance) is the opportunity to learn in the first place. These studies have important implications for abating the current child and adolescent mental health crisis and scaling effective school mental health services. If we are to scale efforts to implement effective practices, we must also scale efforts to increase learning and reduce forgetting among people who are responsible for providing services. This is quite challenging in the field of school mental health, where a widespread and increasing shortage of mental health providers (see Chap. 1, this volume) is further exacerbated by provider turnover rates that have historically exceed 50% (Aarons & Sawitzky, 2006; Aarons et al., 2009; Glisson et al., 2006) and are on the rise (Sklar et al., 2021). The US government and professional organizations are responding to this crisis by both attempting to increase the volume of professionals and re-regulating historically protected services. The latter most notably instantiated in the American Psychological Association's 2024 shift to begin accrediting Master's level programs (historically only reserved for Ph.D. programs) and reconsidering state licensing recommendations; both perhaps are a nod towards shifting the professional practice of psychology to providers with fewer credentials and less formal training. Similar trends are seen in other behavioral health professions, wherein re-regulation is trending towards deploying providers with fewer credentials and less training (e.g., see Oregon's Behavioral Health Workforce white paper; Scheyer et al., 2019). While such efforts will reduce the shortage of school mental health providers, these trends will likely result in a workforce that has less formal training and, as such, will require more on-the-job support and ongoing professional development. Taken together, these trends point towards a clear need to create sustainable training infrastructure that is capable of providing on-demand needs-based training that is easily accessible and germane to school mental health work. Just-in-time training (JITT) is one example of a training innovation that is useful in both increasing the efficiency of learning and reducing forgetting, thereby increasing the scalability of school mental health services.

This chapter describes JITT as a catalyst for scaling effective school mental health. JITT is an on-demand training experience that only includes what is necessary, when it is necessary, to promote competent service delivery for specific tasks. JITT can be used as a supplement to formal training or as opportunities to develop new skills. The key distinguishing features of JITT relative to other training formats (e.g., workshop style; or semester courses) are accessibility and on-demand nature of the training opportunities; they are rendered "just in time." In the sections that follow, we provide examples from other fields, including nursing, medicine, and industry wherein JITT improves efficiency, reduces errors in services, and increases the performance of providers. We provide suggestions for incorporating JITT into efforts to scale effective school-mental health and provide examples and lessons learned from engineering JITT for paraprofessional mentors who support students with behavior problems. Finally, we review key considerations in designing and evaluating JITT.

6.2 Applications of Just-in-Time Training

Just-in-time training (JITT) has emerged as a valuable approach in various professional domains, offering targeted and immediate learning interventions. Medical disciplines were early adopters of JITT. For example, using checklists in healthcare settings has demonstrated efficacy in enhancing services and mitigating morbidity and mortality rates (Weiser et al., 2010). Checklists are one example, perhaps the simplest, of on-demand learning experiences that only include what is necessary, when it is necessary, to promote competent service delivery. While checklists are great prompts for remembering procedural steps, they represent one facet of the multifaceted realm of on-demand learning experiences. Indeed, JITTs on the use of supplemental instructional videos, such as splinting and casting techniques, appear to be effective tools for reducing errors and increasing competency among healthcare professionals (Mehrpour et al., 2013; Wang et al., 2016). Leveraging JITT, medical students can effectively manage their practice time by using instructional videos as resources to address uncertainties about specific task components (Mehrpour et al., 2013). JITT has also been used to help empower medical students in responding to discriminatory comments from patients. For example, following a workshop focused on navigating patients' discriminatory statements, medical students expressed an increased likelihood of responding appropriately to discriminatory comments (Alexander et al., 2021). Moreover, JITT was an important tool during the coronavirus disease 2019 (COVID-19) pandemic. A number of hospitals implemented a JITT program to enhance the preparedness of nursing and hospital staff for effectively managing an increase in critically ill patients and acquiring competencies in disaster medicine (e.g., Duffy & Vergara, 2021; Ragazzoni et al., 2021; Wei et al., 2021; Zucco et al., 2023).

Although medical disciplines were early adopters of JITT, the use of JITT has quickly spread to other fields. During the COVID-19 pandemic, many therapists needed to switch from providing in-person therapy to teletherapy (Sampaio et al., 2021), yet they lacked comprehensive training necessary to effectively conduct teletherapy (Perry et al., 2020). This led to researchers creating accessible JITT resources focused on best practices for delivering effective care to a diverse spectrum of patients during this time (Sampaio et al., 2021). The use of JITT has also been adopted by the military. For example, Saul et al. (2023) used JITTs to increase mental toughness in basic training programs for Navy recruits. In this study, Navy recruits were randomly assigned to supplemental JITTs in mental toughness, which were brief 10-min training experiences on mindfulness, progressive muscle relaxation, and effective self-talk immediately before physical fitness and swim qualification examinations. Those who received the JITTs showed statistically significantly higher graduation rates than those who did not receive the JITT. Saul et al. (2023) study demonstrates the value of JITT in situations that might be mentally and emotionally taxing.

The applicability of JITT extends beyond traditional professional domains into paraprofessionals or lay helpers. For example, providing JITTs to lay helpers (e.g., staff of helping organizations, community volunteers, graduate students) in the immediate aftermath of a disaster on topics such as psychological first aid and common stress reactions can increase the capacity of mental health providers in affected areas (Horn et al., 2019; Wang et al., 2021; Young et al., 2006). This proactive approach aims to enhance survivors' psychological well-being by offering timely support and guidance. JITT programs can also be incorporated into youth mentoring programs to equip volunteer mentors with immediate guidance on how to effectively work with youth identified as having behavioral, emotional, and/or academic difficulties. JITT can provide mentors with essential skills, helping to address the mental health service gap among youth (McQuillin et al., 2019).

6.3   When Might Just-in-Time Training Help Scale Effective School Mental Health?

School mental health professionals use data to make decisions, implement universal prevention efforts, provide tiered therapeutic and support services, collaborate within and between disciplines, and coordinate systems of care in complex and ever-changing environments, among a myriad of other important tasks. Yet increasingly many mental health professionals are entering the workforce with fewer credentials, less training, and less supervised experience (Barnett et al., 2018). Similarly, we increasingly expect teachers, administrators, and other non-traditional providers to support school mental health efforts. Each of these changing circumstances benefits from easily accessible on-demand training content that is designed to transfer specific skills related to modern school mental health efforts. We propose three priority areas that may be particularly important to leverage JITT to scale effective school mental health: (1) supporting changes in school systems, (2) tasks that are prone to error, and (3) low probability events that are consequential or high risk.

6.3.1 Leveraging Just-in-Time Training in the Context of Systems Change

Like most complex systems, the only constant in school systems is change: changing administrations, staff turnover, changes in best practice, new programs, new challenges, innovations in science, etc. While change often presents new opportunities to advance the efforts of school mental health, systems change also involves a substantial amount of energy, time, and resources for onboarding and training personnel in these changes. Leveraging JITT in the context of such changes may present opportunities to increase efficiency and performance within school systems.

An example of this can be found in the South Carolina School Behavioral Health Academy (SC SBHA), which is an on-demand learning management and training system developed by the University of South Carolina in partnership with the South Carolina Department of Health and Human Services (SC DHHS). The SC SBHA was developed in response to two significant changes in school systems beginning in 2022: (1) the surge of demand for mental health services in the wake of the COVID-19 pandemic and (2) SC DHHS policy changes designed to dramatically increase the number of mental health clinicians providing services within schools. These changes resulted in two parallel needs: (1) the need to scale effective mental health services to meet the demand and (2) the need to onboard new mental health clinicians who were beginning (many for the first time) to provide services within the context of school systems. The SC SBHA was a form of JITT designed to fulfill these needs.

The SC SBHA offers free, on-demand, and fully asynchronous training opportunities on the fundamentals of Multi-Tiered Systems of Support (MTSS) and Interconnected Systems Framework (ISF) for school personnel in the state of South Carolina. The goal of the SC SBHA is to enhance knowledge and competent practice for everyone who works to support the social, emotional, and behavioral needs of students in South Carolina by leveraging knowledge on best-practice and translating that knowledge to pragmatic screening, prevention, tiered intervention, and progress monitoring activities. The SC SBHA includes video tutorials and examples from dozens of school mental health experts across the country on a wide range of topics, as well as interactive learning media. Importantly, the coursework in the SC SBHA is accessible at any time, even following the completion of courses, and learners can re-enter the system to review key concepts or strategies on-demand. In addition to the online asynchronous content, the SC SBHA offers synchronous tele-coaching to school districts on how to use the SC SBHA to improve MTSS functioning in order to scale effective school mental health efforts.

The SC SBHA offers continuing education credits and certificates of competency for completing courses, which are designed to accommodate a range of school personnel. For example, the course "All Hands on Deck" is designed for anyone who works in school, focusing on school-wide wellness promotion and mental health stigma reduction. As the name would suggest, this course emphasizes *all* school personnel who interact with students, ranging from transportation workers (e.g., bus drivers) to principals. In contrast, the course, "Growing Your Tier 3 Supports," is focused on improving intensive interventions (i.e., Tier 3, see Chap. 2, this volume) within the context of MTSS and ISF. This course's audience are those responsible for providing more intensive interventions including special education teachers, board certified behavior analysts, existing school clinicians, and those who are transitioning to become school clinicians from community or private organizations. Collectively, the SC SBHA is an example of leveraging learning technology to provide on-demand training experiences during a rapidly changing school mental health infrastructure. More information on the SC SBHA can be found at scsbha.org.

6.3.2 Reducing Errors Through Just-in-Time Training

Using JITT to reduce errors may also be a fruitful endeavor. Simple reminders of learned skills—things like checklists—are often enough to prevent errors in many tasks. Evidence for checklists' capacity to reduce errors in practice is precisely why surgeons across the globe use tools like the World Health Organization (WHO) Surgical Safety Checklist (WHO, 2009). Yet, checklists are likely to be helpful only to the extent providers have mastery over the tasks prompted in each step of the checklist, and will be insufficient to the extent that providers lack competency. As efforts to scale school mental health increasingly turn to task-shifting, or the redistribution of tasks from professionals to workers with fewer credentials or less training, it is likely that errors will increase unless they are effectively managed (McQuillin et al., 2019). In these cases, JITT focused on improving competency and reducing errors may be helpful. For example, and as will be discussed below in the Sect. 6.5 case example, JITT that uses video examples (and counter examples of errors) can be helpful in reducing the likelihood of errors when lay helpers provide evidence-based counseling approaches, like Motivational Interviewing (MI). Similar strategies could be used across the range of tasks performed in MTSS teams.

Effective school mental health efforts, for instance, require a diverse cast of characters that are charged with working together to review data, make decisions, and provide competent services, among other tasks. At each of these levels, there are risks for errors. As mentioned in Chap. 1, (this volume) well-functioning teams are the foundation of effective MTSS. Yet, in many cases, these teams do not function as intended. For example, Crone et al. (2016) recorded and coded the efforts of "data-based decision making" teams in middle schools and found that the teams rarely reviewed actionable data for student behavior concerns, and in the majority of cases (~66%), the teams did not make actionable decisions. Moreover, it was even rarer for the teams to follow up and adjust decisions after they were made. This research is helpful in identifying potential opportunities to reduce errors and improve functioning in MTSS using JITT. This research also reifies the importance of on-demand training opportunities like the SC SBHA mentioned above given the range of backgrounds and formal education experiences of team members. School systems and researchers would be wise to similarly analyze error prone domains of school mental health services and match these with implementation supports like JITT.

6.3.3   Low Probability But Consequential Events

Finally, we suggest JITT may be particularly important for events that are low probability but consequential. These so-called "black swan events," unpredictable events that have large and consequential impacts, include environmental disasters, critical incidents at school (e.g., school shootings) or in communities (e.g., community violence), among others. Some of the aforementioned examples of JITT were developed to respond to similar events, including JITTs designed to provide universal mental health first aid following disasters and JITT designed to help clinicians navigate the transition to teletherapy after COVID-19 lockdowns. The common denominator of these events is their unpredictability and their impact on system functioning.

Similar to the first two priority areas (i.e., changes within school systems and error prone events), low probability but consequential events create a need to rapidly and efficiently prepare helpers to respond in an effective manner while also navigating risks for error. Such events carry additional risks because they are not routine, workers may not have experience or formal training in responding to these events, and new workers, including lay helpers, may be recruited to help respond. Examples include how schools navigate and respond to tragic critical incidents in schools, like school shootings or the death of students. These tragic events often leave school helpers desperate to support students, yet evidence would suggest that some helping efforts carry risks and can even be harmful. In a review of iatrogenic interventions in schools, Raines et al. (2010) describe common but harmful approaches to responding to tragic school events. For example, Critical Incident Stress Debriefing—universal debriefings and discussions of negative emotions with students following a traumatic event—can *increase* posttraumatic stress disorder symptoms. In these circumstances, school personnel may consider JITT as an opportunity to share knowledge on best-practices to reduce the likelihood that school personnel use contraindicated interventions.

6.4   Factors That Influence the Success of Just-in-Time Training

6.4.1   Clear, Behavior-Based, Learning Objectives

While the simple act of implementing just-in-time training (JITT) for school mental health professionals may increase provider effectiveness, there are several factors that influence just *how* successful these training opportunities will be at reducing forgetting over time. The first such factor is the presence of clear criteria for competency demonstration. To ensure learner success, those interested in developing JITT should start with the end in mind. In other words, the first element of a JITT should be clearly defined learning objectives that explain specific criteria for competency demonstration. These objectives will ideally include the main takeaways of the training, written in terms of what learners will be *able to do* after participating in the training. Clearly defining criteria for competency demonstration will allow training developers to create a learning experience that most adequately meets these goals. Presenting course objectives to learners enhances skill transfer by allowing learners to more clearly understand what is expected of them (Taylor et al., 2005). Research evidence from a meta-analysis of 53 studies investigating factors that impact the usefulness of JITT found that evaluating learners based on behaviors rather than learning (i.e., what they actually do in practice rather than what they know how to do) moderated the success of training (Arthur et al., 1998). With this in mind, it is possible that behaviorally focused learning objectives may result in greater levels of skill transfer than cognitive-focused objectives. For instance, *"Counselors will avoid evaluative judgements when clients disclose substance use behavior and instead use reflective statements and affirmations"* may be a more concrete and transferrable learning objective than *"Counselors will understand the importance of empathy in conversations about substance use."*

6.4.2 Juxtaposition of Desired and Undesired Behaviors

Like the example above, in addition to clearly communicating how learners *should* behave at the end of a training, research indicates that it is also important to clearly communicate how they *should not* behave. Juxtaposing the intended training outcome or target behavior with an example of a poorly executed outcome or behavior is another way to increase training effectiveness. Trainings that provide both positive and negative examples or models of desired behaviors for learners to follow (i.e., *mixed-models*) tend to be more effective than training that only provides positive models (Taylor et al., 2005). Providing both positive and negative examples can help facilitate skill transfer by helping learners "unlearn" undesirable behaviors. Providing a range of examples has also been found to increase learners' generalization of principles from the training to the real-life context (Baldwin, 1992). For example, a study by Hart et al. (2024; discussed further below) included the use of juxtaposition in the creation of JITT videos for paraprofessional's practice of Motivational Interviewing (MI) with adolescents. Specifically, one of the key challenges of helping young people change their behaviors is avoiding something MI researchers call the *righting reflex*, or the reflexive tendency of helpers to offer unsolicited advice, provide suggestions, or warn young people, collectively; these behaviors attempt to "right" a perceived wrong using verbal behaviors. These behaviors typically backfire, and disrupt the helping relationship, making it less likely that young people will change their behavior. In order to reinforce the importance of avoiding the righting reflex, Hart et al. (2024) created video examples that included the desired response (e.g., accurate expressions of empathy or open-ended questions) with those of undesired responses (e.g., providing unsolicited advice or warning the client).

6.4.3 Attending to Cognitive and Affective Appraisals of Training

According to Kirpatrick's Training Model (1959, 1987), training and learning programs should be evaluated not only based on their results, but also learners' (1) reactions to the training, (2) level of learning, (3) behaviors following the training, and (4) results. Learners' reactions to training encompasses their impressions of or feelings about the training, whereas their level of learning assesses the knowledge or skills they acquire from the training. Behaviors refer to how learners perform at the *point-of-performance* (i.e., when the desired behavior would be routinely demonstrated). Results indicate the overall effectiveness of these behaviors and, in turn, effectiveness of the training in attaining program outcomes (i.e., successfully fulfilling training objectives or overarching program goals). With this in mind, the learner's own thoughts, feelings, and behavioral reactions to the JITT are also likely to influence its effectiveness. Intentionally monitoring outcomes across each of these levels can ensure that learners are getting the most out of JITT. To illustrate this, one study comparing training and support models for school- and community-based mentoring programs found that mentors who participated in a program that featured an ongoing or enhanced training model (i.e., those who were provided with "booster trainings" periodically in addition to a traditional pre-match training) reacted more positively than those who were not provided with ongoing support. Specifically, mentors who received JITT reported feeling more supported by their program, felt that their training was more valuable, and expressed intent to continue providing the service as compared to those in a program without enhanced training or support (McQuillin et al., 2015). These differences in perceived support, training value, and intent to continue mentoring also predicted increased relationship satisfaction between the mentor and mentee, suggesting that not only did the training make mentors feel better and engage in more mentoring, but also made them more effective at mentoring. With this in mind, considering multiple layers of evaluation that emphasize both learner reactions and knowledge transfer can ensure maximum effectiveness of JITT.

6.4.4   Carefully Considering the Timing of Training

Another factor that influences the success of JITT is *how closely* the training is aligned to the point of performance. Consistent with Ebbinghaus's (2013) early findings regarding learning and forgetting, individuals are less likely to remember what they have learned the longer time passes. Indeed, research findings from Arthur and colleagues' (1998) meta analysis found that skill retention decreases as the period of time between the JITT and the point of performance or practice increases. They observed that skill loss could be observed as soon as less than 1 day from the point of training, further emphasizing the importance of closely aligning the training with the point of performance. With this in mind, implementing JITT as close to the point of performance as possible ensures maximum usefulness for learners.

Similarly, providing learners with cues at the point of performance can increase the usefulness of JITT. These cues can take many forms ranging in complexity from supplementary video tutorials to checklists. Regardless of their specific formats, these cues serve as additional reminders regarding what learners have learned. The literature on learning indicates that additional prompts or cues can help facilitate the retrieval of information that one has previously learned and, in turn, decrease skill decay. For example, one research study of JITT in healthcare compared whether there were significant differences in how well medical students could apply splints to bodily injuries based on whether they watched a brief supplemental video tutorial beforehand (Mehrpour et al., 2013). All medical students received the same initial training (i.e., a 90-min lecture). The researchers found that the students who had access to a memory cue performed significantly better than those who did not have access to this cue. These findings have been replicated with similar outcomes in another study that also examined the effectiveness of a brief video tutorial cue for physicians when applying splints, who received their initial training in a small workshop setting (Wang et al., 2016). Another study found that a visual cue in the form of a checklist provided on a bandage dressing package significantly increased nurses' confidence and competence in applying the dressing to patients (Kent, 2010). Specifically, 88% of the nurses who had access to the visual cue were able to apply the dressing correctly, whereas none of the nurses who used the traditional bandage packaging (i.e., without the visual cue) were able to apply it correctly. Nurses who had access to the checklist also reported they felt much more confident in their abilities to apply the dressings. Although the simple presence of a checklist or other form of cue can be helpful, one study specifically examining the effectiveness of computer versus paper checklists found that learners who used computer-based checklists performed significantly faster and more proficiently than those who used a paper checklist. This indicates that leaning into technology for these additional cues may be a valuable avenue for school mental health professionals (Seagull et al., 2007).

6.5   A Case Example of Applying JITT to Expand School Mental Health Supports

As mentioned in Chap. 1 of this volume, efforts to scale effective school mental health will depend on expanding access to supports beyond traditional professional providers. One such example of these efforts is the use of volunteer mentors to provide emotional and behavioral supports (McQuillin et al., 2022). However, there are risks involved in encouraging lay helpers to provide support to vulnerable students, and some studies have shown iatrogenic outcomes when volunteer mentors are poorly trained (McQuillin et al., 2011). A critical factor in fostering safe and effective mentoring relationships is ongoing training and support (McQuillin & Lyons, 2021). With proper training and support, it appears that volunteer mentors can produce positive student outcomes in social, emotional, and academic areas (McQuillin & McDaniel, 2021).

A case example of this can be found in a series of studies evaluating Brief Instrumental School-Based Mentoring (BISBM), which is a time limited (i.e., single semester), goal focused volunteer mentoring program for middle school students intended to improve social, emotional, academic, and behavioral functioning. Mentors in BISBM are trained in the counseling style of Motivational Interviewing (MI) and follow a modular curriculum designed to help middle school students select and pursue goals related to school functioning. Mentors also spend time with mentees in relationship building activities and unstructured recreation time (e.g., basketball, board games) during or after school hours. The hope of BISBM is that support services for students in need could be expanded by leveraging volunteer lay helpers to provide services. In theory, this could effectively expand access to services.

An early study of BISBM found that students who were randomly assigned to receive a mentor showed *decreased* reading grades and null outcomes on a range of other measures (McQuillin et al., 2011). In this study, students assigned a mentor performed worse than students who experienced school as usual on average. After the fact, researchers found that mentors in the program (mostly college students) were not performing the key mentoring behaviors (e.g., supporting youth autonomy when setting goals), were using strategies that were unlikely to be effective (e.g., arguing with mentees about their grades or behavior), and were not following the guided curriculum (e.g., only engaging in unstructured recreation time). Put simply, it appeared that mentors had forgotten or were not using the training that they received a month prior to being matched with their mentee. These errors were consequential, resulting in poorer school performance for those who received a mentor. However, researchers later revised the program to include proactive support (i.e., check-ins immediately prior to mentoring) and JITT videos that reinforced effective mentoring behaviors and actively discouraged ineffective or potentially harmful behaviors. Subsequent evaluations of this revised program resulted in improved effectiveness across a range of student outcomes, including academic, emotional, and behavioral domains (see McQuillin et al., 2019 for a review of the revisions and evaluations). It appears that with such ongoing JITT and proactive support, BISBM can help support social, emotional, academic, and behavioral outcomes of youth who show high levels of impairment (McQuillin & McDaniel, 2021). Thus, the safety and effectiveness of this service, which uses lay helpers as the primary provider, depends substantially on the structure of training and support systems, primarily the use of JITT.

A recent study of BISBM by Hart et al. (under review), mentioned above in Sect. 6.4.2, tested the effectiveness of the JITT on mentors' knowledge of, attitudes about, and skills in Motivational Interviewing (MI). In this study, volunteer mentors working with middle school students were randomly assigned to one of two conditions. The first condition (i.e., the control group) involved pre-match training (i.e., a pre-program training seminar to help mentors prepare for the program) in MI as well as ongoing proactive supervision throughout the course of the mentoring relationship. The second condition (i.e., the treatment group) received the same training and proactive supervision as the control group in addition to mentors being asked to watch 3–5 min JITT videos that demonstrated key MI skills as they related to particular sessions in the program immediately prior to the mentoring session. For example, during the first meeting between mentors and mentees, mentors guide mentees through a value card sort activity, wherein mentees identify their top values (e.g., "making my parents proud") and connect these values to their school behavior (e.g., "How do you make your parents proud at school?"). A common error in this activity is that mentors will focus on values that mentees rate as not important, rather than encouraging and discussing the values that mentees rate as important. The JITT video for this session involved a brief didactic explanation of desired behaviors (e.g., open-ended questions, affirmations, reflections, and summaries) as well as juxtaposed undesired behaviors (e.g., arguing) followed by a live action video example of both. This and similar videos were provided to the treatment group mentors throughout the course of the single-semester mentoring intervention, with mentors being prompted to watch the video immediately prior to the session. The researchers found that mentors who watched the brief JITT videos showed improvements in MI knowledge, attitudes, and skills. Thus, incorporating JITT may be one way to improve the effectiveness of school behavioral health efforts that involve lay helpers or paraprofessionals.

6.6   Conclusion

Efforts to scale effective school mental health will face challenges equipping an evolving workforce to sustain evidence-based practices in ever-changing systems. Forgetting or failing to implement best practices is one significant threat to these efforts. Just-in-time training (JITT) is one implementation support that has been shown to be helpful in reducing forgetting, improving the effectiveness of services, reducing the likelihood of errors, and increasing the efficiency of training and support resources. Examples of JITT range from simple efforts, like the inclusion of checklists or brief pre-service videos, to comprehensive learning management systems that are capable of rendering training in best practices on-demand.

School administrators and clinicians may consider leveraging JITT in situations wherein school systems or practices are changing rapidly, in supporting practices that are prone to error, or in responding to unpredictable but consequential events. Researchers in school behavioral health will improve JITT efforts by identifying such situations and testing training models designed to help knowledge and skill retention. An example of this is the aforementioned work by Hart et al. (2024) on testing the knowledge and skill retention of providers following brief video examples and counterexamples of counseling approaches. Similarly, as evidenced in the South Carolina School Behavioral Health Academy (SC SBHA), universities will play a critical role in supporting JITT efforts through partnerships with public entities interested in scaling effective school mental health practices. Finally, JITT presents new opportunities to scale effective practices among helpers that have historically not been involved in the promotion of mental health, including lay helpers, community members, or other school personnel.

References

Aarons, A. G., & Sawitzky, A. C. (2006). Organizational climate partially mediates the effect of culture on work attitudes and staff turnover in mental health services. *Administration and Policy in Mental Health and Mental Health Services Research, 33*(3), 289–301. https://doi.org/10.1007/s10488-006-0039-1

Aarons, G. A., Sommerfeld, D. H., Hecht, D. B., Silovsky, J. F., & Chaffin, M. J. (2009). The impact of evidence-based practice implementation and fidelity monitoring on staff turnover: Evidence for a protective effect. *Journal of Consulting and Clinical Psychology, 77*(2), 270–280. https://doi.org/10.1037/a0013223

Alexander, A., Singh, M., Scott, A., Moreira, R., Atkinson, T., Fissel, R., Tariq, S., & Patil, S. (2021). Empowering medical students to respond to discriminatory comments from patients: A just-in-time training method. *MedEdPublish, 10*(1), 129. https://doi.org/10.15694/mep.2021.000129.1

Arthur, W., Jr., Bennett, W., Jr., Stanush, P. L., & McNelly, T. L. (1998). Factors that influence skill decay and retention: A quantitative review and analysis. *Human Performance, 11*(1), 57–101. https://doi.org/10.1207/s15327043hup1101_3

Baldwin, T. T. (1992). Effects of alternative modeling strategies on outcomes of interpersonal-skills training. *Journal of Applied Psychology, 77*(2), 147–154. https://doi.org/10.1037/0021-9010.77.2.147

Barnett, M. L., Lau, A. S., & Miranda, J. (2018). Lay health worker involvement in evidence-based treatment delivery: A conceptual model to address disparities in care. *Annual Review of Clinical Psychology, 14*, 185–208. https://doi.org/10.1146/annurev-clinpsy-050817-084825

Crone, D. A., Carlson, S. E., Haack, M. K., Kennedy, P. C., Baker, S. K., & Fien, H. (2016). Data-based decision-making teams in middle school: Observations and implications from the middle school intervention project. *Assessment for Effective Intervention, 41*(2), 79–93. https://doi.org/10.1177/1534508415610322

Duffy, J. R., & Vergara, M. A. (2021). Just-in-time training for the use of ICU nurse extenders during COVID-19 pandemic response. *Military Medicine, 186*(2), 40–43. https://doi.org/10.1093/milmed/usab195

Ebbinghaus, H. (2013). Memory: A contribution to experimental psychology. *Annals of Neurosciences, 20*(4), 155–156. https://doi.org/10.5214/ans.0972.7531.200408

Gawande, A. (2010). *Checklist manifesto, the (HB)*. Penguin Group.

Glisson, C., Dukes, D., & Green, P. (2006). The effects of the ARC organizational intervention on caseworker turnover, climate, and culture in children's service systems. *Child Abuse and Neglect, 30*(8), 855–880. https://doi.org/10.1016/j.chiabu.2005.12.010

Hart, M., McQuillin, S. D., Iachini, A., Cooper, D., & Weist, M. (2024). *The efficacy and usability of motivational interviewing just-in-time trainings for youth mentors*. [Manuscript submitted for publication]. Department of Educational Psychology, University of Texas at San Antonio.

Haynes, A. B., Weiser, T. G., Berry, W. R., Lipsitz, S. R., Breizat, A. H. S., Dellinger, E. P., Herbosa, T., Joseph, S., Kibatala, P. L., Lapitan, M. C. M., Merry, A. F., Moorthy, K., Reznick, R. K., Taylor, B., & Gawande, A. A. (2009). A surgical safety checklist to reduce morbidity and mortality in a global population. *New England Journal of Medicine, 360*(5), 491–499. https://doi.org/10.1056/NEJMsa0810119

Horn, R., O'May, F., Esliker, R., Gwaikolo, W., Woensdregt, L., Ruttenberg, L., & Ager, A. (2019). The myth of the 1-day training: The effectiveness of psychosocial support capacity-building during the Ebola outbreak in West Africa. *Global Mental Health, 6*(e5), 1–15. https://doi.org/10.1017/gmh.2019.2

Kent, D. J. (2010). Effects of a just-in-time educational intervention placed on wound dressing packages: A multicenter randomized controlled trial. *Journal of Wound, Ostomy, and Continence Nursing, 37*(6), 609–614. https://doi.org/10.1097/WON.0b013e3181f1826b

Kirkpatrick, D. L. (1959). Techniques for evaluation training programs. *Journal of the American Society of Training Directors, 13*, 21–26.

Kirkpatrick, D. L. (1987). Evaluation of training. In R. L. Craig (Ed.), *Training and development handbook: A guide to human resource development* (pp. 301–319). McGraw-Hill.

Madson, M. B., Loignon, A. C., & Lane, C. (2009). Training in motivational interviewing: A systematic review. *Journal of Substance Abuse Treatment, 36*(1), 101–109. https://doi.org/10.1016/j.jsat.2008.05.005

McQuillin, S. D., & Lyons, M. D. (2021). A national study of mentoring program characteristics and premature match closure: The role of program training and ongoing support. *Prevention Science, 22*, 334–344. https://doi.org/10.1007/s11121-020-01200-9

McQuillin, S. D., & McDaniel, H. L. (2021). Pilot randomized trial of brief school-based mentoring for middle school students with elevated disruptive behavior. *Annals of the New York Academy of Sciences, 1483*(1), 127–141. https://doi.org/10.1111/nyas.14334

McQuillin, S., Smith, B., & Strait, G. (2011). Randomized evaluation of a single semester transitional mentoring program for first year middle school students: A cautionary result for brief, school-based mentoring programs. *Journal of Community Psychology, 39*, 844–859. https://doi.org/10.1002/jcop.20475

McQuillin, S. D., Straight, G. G., & Saeki, E. (2015). Program support and value of training in mentors' satisfaction and anticipated continuation of school-based mentoring relationships. *Mentoring & Tutoring: Partnership in Learning, 23*(2), 133–148. https://doi.org/10.1080/13611267.2015.1047630

McQuillin, S. D., Lyons, M. D., Becker, K. D., Hart, M. J., & Cohen, K. (2019). Strengthening and expanding child services in low resource communities: The role of task-shifting and just-in-time training. *American Journal of Community Psychology, 63*(3–4), 355–365. https://doi.org/10.1002/ajcp.12314

McQuillin, S. D., Hagler, M. A., Werntz, A., & Rhodes, J. E. (2022). Paraprofessional youth mentoring: A framework for integrating youth mentoring with helping institutions and professions. *American Journal of Community Psychology, 69*(1–2), 201–220. https://doi.org/10.1002/ajcp.12546

Mehrpour, S. R., Aghamirsalim, M., Motamedi, S. M. K., Larijani, F. A., & Sorbi, R. (2013). A supplemental video teaching tool enhances splinting skills. *Clinical Orthopaedics and Related Research, 471*(2), 649–665. https://doi.org/10.1007/s11999-012-2638-3

Miller, W. R., Yahne, C. E., Moyers, T. B., Martinez, J., & Pirritano, M. (2004). A randomized trial of methods to help clinicians learn motivational interviewing. *Journal of Consulting and Clinical Psychology, 72*(6), 1050–1062. https://doi.org/10.1037/0022-006x.72.6.1050

Perry, K., Gold, S., & Shearer, E. M. (2020). Identifying and addressing mental health providers' perceived barriers to clinical video telehealth utilization. *Journal of Clinical Psychology, 76*(6), 1125–1134. https://doi.org/10.1002/jclp.22770

Ragazzoni, L., Barco, A., Echeverri, L., Conti, A., Linty, M., Caviglia, M., Merlo, F., Martini, D., Pirisi, A., Weinstein, E., Barone-Adesi, F., & Della Corte, F. (2021). Just-in-time training in a tertiary referral hospital during the COVID-19 pandemic in Italy. *Academic Medicine, 96*(3), 336–339. https://doi.org/10.1097/ACM.0000000000003575

Sampaio, M., Haro, M. V. N., De Sousa, B., Melo, W. V., & Hoffman, H. G. (2021). Therapists make the switch to telepsychology to safely continue treating their patients during the COVID-19 pandemic: Virtual reality telepsychology may be next. *Frontiers in Virtual Reality, 1*, 1–17. https://doi.org/10.3389/frvir.2020.576421

Saul, K. M., Young, M. D., Siddiqi, J. M., & Hirsch, D. A. (2023). Developing a mental toughness program for basic military training. *Military Psychology, 36*(2), 203–213. https://doi.org/10.1080/08995605.2023.2167467

Scheyer, K., Gilchrist, E. C., Muther, J., Hemeida, S., & Wong, S. L. (2019). *Recruitment and retention recommendations for Oregon's behavioral health workforce* [White paper]. Farley Health Policy Center. https://www.oregon.gov/oha/HPA/ANALYTICS/HealthCareWorkforceReporting/2019-04-Recruitment-Retention-Recs-Oregon-BH-Workforce.pdf

Schwalbe, C. S., Oh, H. Y., & Zweben, A. (2014). Sustaining motivational interviewing: A meta-analysis of training studies. *Society for the Study of Addiction, 109*(8), 1287–1294. https://doi.org/10.1111/add.12558

Seagull, F. J., Ho, D., Radcliffe, J., Xiao, Y., Hu, P., & Mackenzie, C. F. (2007). Just-in-time training for medical emergencies: Computer versus paper checklists for a tracheal intubation task. *Proceedings of the Human Factors and Ergonomics Society Annual Meeting, 51*(11), 725–729. https://doi.org/10.1177/154193120705101126

Sibley, M. H., Bickman, L., Coxe, S. J., Graziano, P. A., & Martin, P. (2021). Community implementation of MI-enhanced behavior therapy for adolescent ADHD: Linking fidelity to effectiveness. *Behavior Therapy, 52*(4), 847–860. https://doi.org/10.1016/j.beth.2020.10.007

Sklar, M., Ehrhart, M. G., & Aarons, G. A. (2021). COVID-related work changes, burnout, and turnover intentions in mental health providers: A moderated mediation analysis. *Psychiatric Rehabilitation Journal, 44*(3), 219–228. https://doi.org/10.1037/prj0000480

Smith, J., Carpenter, K., Amrhein, P., Brooks, A., Levin, D., Schreiber, E., Travaglini, L., Hu, M. N., & Nunes, E. (2012). Training substance abuse clinicians in motivational interviewing using live supervision via teleconferencing. *Journal of Consulting and Clinical Psychology, 80*(3), 450–464. https://doi.org/10.1037/a0028176

Taylor, P. J., Russ-Eft, D. F., & Chan, D. W. L. (2005). A meta-analytic review of behavior modeling training. *Journal of Applied Psychology, 90*(4), 692–709. https://doi.org/10.1037/0021-9010.90.4.692

Wang, V., Cheng, Y. T., & Liu, D. (2016). Improving education: Just-in-time splinting video. *The Clinical Teacher, 13*(3), 183–186. https://doi.org/10.1111/tct.12394

Wang, L., Norman, I., Xiao, T., Li, Y., & Leamy, M. (2021). Psychological first aid training: A scoping review of its application, outcomes and implementation. *International Journal of Environmental Research and Public Health, 8*(9), 4594. https://doi.org/10.3390/ijerph18094594

Wei, E. K., Long, T., & Katz, M. H. (2021). Nine lessons learned from the COVID-19 pandemic for improving hospital care and health care delivery. *JAMA Internal Medicine, 181*(9), 1161–1163. https://doi.org/10.1001/jamainternmed.2021.4237

Weiser, T. G., Haynes, A. B., Lashoher, A., Dziekan, G., Boorman, D. J., Berry, W. R., & Gawande, A. A. (2010). Perspectives in quality: Designing the WHO surgical safety checklist. *International Journal for Quality in Health Care, 22*(5), 365–370. https://doi.org/10.1093/intqhc/mzq039

World Health Organization. (2009). *Surgical safety checklist*. https://iris.who.int/bitstream/handle/10665/44186/9789241598590_eng_Checklist.pdf?sequence=2&isAllowed=y

Young, B. H., Ruzek, J. I., Wong, M., Salzer, M. S., & Naturale, A. J. (2006). Disaster mental health training: Guidelines, considerations, and recommendations. In E. C. Ritchie, P. J. Watson, & M. J. Friedman (Eds.), *Interventions following mass violence and disasters: Strategies for mental health practice* (pp. 54–79). The Guilford Press.

Zucco, L., Chen, M. J., Levy, N., Obeidat, S. S., Needham, M. J., Hyatt, A., Keane, J. R., Pollard, R. J., Mitchell, J. D., & Ramachandran, S. K. (2023). Just-in-time in situ simulation training as a preparedness measure for the perioperative care of COVID-19 patients. *Simulation in Healthcare: The Journal of the Society for Simulation in Healthcare, 18*(2), 90–99. https://doi.org/10.1097/SIH.0000000000000635

Chapter 7
Scaling School Mental Health with Single Session Interventions

Katherine A. Cohen, Jenna Y. Sung, Megan L. McCormick, and Jessica L. Schleider

7.1 Scaling School Mental Health with Single Session Interventions

The child and adolescent mental health crisis is complex, encompassing financial and geographic barriers to care, a shortage of trained providers, personal and systemic stigma, restrictions on youth autonomy, and numerous other concerns identified and discussed in-depth by previous authors (Kazdin, 2017; Radez et al., 2022). It follows that the solution to these concerns must be similarly complex, incorporating a broad array of strategies. In addition to strengthening traditional methods of mental health service delivery, new avenues for ameliorating the mental health crisis must be explored to build a comprehensive and variegated system of support (Gruber et al., 2021; Kazdin, 2019). In this chapter, we introduce one potential avenue: school-based single session interventions.

K. A. Cohen (✉) · J. L. Schleider
Department of Medical Social Sciences, Northwestern University Feinberg School of Medicine, Chicago, IL, USA
e-mail: katie.cohen@northwestern.edu

J. Y. Sung
Department of Psychology, Stony Brook University, Stony Brook, NY, USA

M. L. McCormick
MedStar Georgetown Center for Wellbeing in School Environments, Washington, DC, USA

7.1.1 Single Session Interventions (SSIs)

SSIs are defined as "structured programs that intentionally involve only one visit or encounter with a clinic, provider, or program (Schleider et al., 2020a, p. 1)." Intentionality is crucial in this definition; an intervention limited to one session due to dropout, or an intervention designed to be multi-sessioned that is not delivered in full due to resource constraints, would not be considered an SSI. Instead, the SSI approach encourages intervention developers and/or providers to consider how meaningful change can occur in a single encounter. This compels the intervention developer and/or provider to critically consider what mechanism they should target based on what has demonstrated efficacy for a particular problem, population, or setting. This is not to suggest that an individual cannot complete multiple SSIs, each targeting different mechanisms, or repeat the same SSI multiple times. Rather, the SSI approach suggests that if only one encounter or intervention is feasible to implement, it can still have a positive impact.

A common misconception surrounding SSIs is that they are intended to replace longer-term therapy with trained providers. SSIs are not a panacea, they are not appropriate for all mental health concerns, nor should they replace therapy. Rather, they are one avenue for scaling mental health services in the current landscape, which is characterized by the fact that most youth with mental health needs will not receive any treatment. However, we also caution against viewing SSIs as inherently inferior to long-term interventions. That is, a misconception surrounding SSIs is that it is not possible to see long-term improvements in mental health outcomes after only one session. In fact, meta-analytic findings suggest that SSIs can lead to reductions in mental health concerns that are comparable in effect size to longer-term interventions; for example, SSIs targeting anxiety show an overall effect size of Hedges $g = 0.56$ at post-intervention (Schleider & Weisz, 2017), while interventions targeting anxiety that are 12–14 sessions long show an overall effect size of Hedges $g = 0.61$ at post-intervention (Weisz et al., 2017). Other work suggests that positive benefits from a 30-min SSI can be seen as far as 9-months post-intervention (Schleider & Weisz, 2018). There may be a perception that the longer a treatment is, the more effective it must be, yet there is evidence in the reverse: meta-analyses have found that greater intervention time is associated with smaller positive effects (Öst & Ollendick, 2017; Weisz et al., 2017).

The appeal of SSIs is in their ease of implementation combined with their evidence of efficacy. As a result, research on SSIs has rapidly increased in quantity and variety in the last decade. SSIs have been designed to target a diverse range of concerns including anxiety, depression, conduct problems, and substance use (McDanal et al., 2022; Schleider & Weisz, 2017). Some are designed to be self-administered while others are provider-delivered, with providers ranging from trained mental health clinicians to lay workers (Hart et al., 2022; Schleider et al., 2020b; Shen et al., 2023). Many are web-based or delivered via telehealth, while others take place in-person (Schleider et al., 2020b, 2021; Sung et al., 2023). When considering

SSIs designed to ameliorate mental health concerns in children and adolescents, one setting is critical to examine in further detail: schools.

7.2 School-Based Mental Health Services

Schools are ideal settings to deliver mental health interventions. Schools are already one of the most common settings where youth access mental health services (Duong et al., 2021). In addition, teachers are often the first adult to identify that a child is struggling with their mental health due to their level of contact with students and their responsibility to monitor students' academic and behavioral progress (Dimitropoulos et al., 2022). Further, the simple fact that students are required to attend school and are provided with methods to be transported there suggests that when school-based services are offered, barriers to access related to location and transportation are minimized. Schools are particularly well equipped to facilitate access to services for populations that are typically underserved by the mental health system, such as children in low resource households, children in rural areas, or children whose parents are undocumented immigrants (Fazel et al., 2014; Love et al., 2019). From a public health perspective, schools are one of the only settings where the majority of a population (i.e., children) is found in one place, meaning it is ripe for universal prevention efforts (Herrenkohl, 2019). Particularly for interventions where a major component is psychoeducation, presenting the content in a school setting amidst other learning initiatives is intuitive. The potential benefits of school-based mental health services are manifold; however, problems can arise if the limitations of the school setting are not considered (Baker et al., 2021; Lyon, 2021).

Schools are limited in resources, including both time and money. Teachers report that the curriculums they are required to teach contain more material than they can realistically cover during the school year, requiring them to utilize every minute of instruction they can (Organisation for Economic Cooperation and Development, 2020). Suggesting that schools dedicate multiple days or weeks toward implementing a mental health program may not be realistic. Further, teachers and school staff describe feeling overworked and are at risk of experiencing secondary traumatic stress and compassion fatigue (Ormiston et al., 2022; Robinson et al., 2023). Programs that require teachers or other school personnel to spend extensive time and mental capacity undergoing training in how to facilitate/administer the program could be seen as another burden. Relatedly, schools face financial limitations. Schools may not be capable of dedicating funds toward expanding or improving mental health programs; approximately half of school staff list "inadequate funding" as a reason they cannot effectively provide mental health care to students (Panchal et al., 2022). The combination of these concerns suggests that school-based mental health interventions may be optimally acceptable if they are brief, demand minimal resources, and do not require lengthy staff training. Thus, we introduce school-based SSIs as a potential solution.

7.3 School-Based SSIs

SSIs delivered in schools may provide an effective method to reduce mental health concerns by allowing for wide dissemination of psychoeducational and skill-building content, expanding access to care for students who would not or cannot receive lengthier services, and reducing the demand for services from trained providers, thereby possibly reducing burnout. Below we discuss the potential audiences for school-based SSIs, examples from the literature of school-based SSIs, and the role of SSIs in multitiered systems of support.

7.3.1 Multiple Audiences

School-based SSIs may be designed for students, school staff, or other individuals within the school system. For example, student-directed SSIs may address transdiagnostic mechanisms lying beneath internalizing symptomatology, such as hopelessness or loneliness (Barkus & Badcock, 2019; Castellanos-Ryan et al., 2016; Eccles et al., 2020). Several such SSIs are freely available online (https://www.schleiderlab.org), and there is evidence to support that they reduce mental health concerns among youth (Dobias et al., 2021; Schleider et al., 2020b; Shen et al., 2023). While previous research on these SSIs has used digital methods to recruit youth (i.e., social media), schools provide an ideal context to make youth aware and encourage them to complete these interventions. Additionally, schools provide a context for following up with youth who may have indicated greater risk or who see no positive changes after the intervention.

There is a small literature on already-existing school-based SSIs targeting mental health or wellbeing in students. In a systematic review of brief school-based mental health interventions, several SSIs showed evidence of efficacy (Cohen et al., 2024). For example, *The Shamiri Intervention* is a digital, self-guided intervention that teaches youth about growth mindset in one 60-min session. In a trial with 103 students in a secondary school in Kenya, participants in Shamiri had greater reductions in depression, as measured by the PHQ-8, at a 2-week follow-up compared to participants in an attention-matched control condition (Osborn et al., 2020). Another example is the *Enhanced Psychological Mindset Session for Adolescents*, a digital, self-guided intervention that teaches youth about acceptance and self-compassion in one 30-min session. In a trial with 80 highschoolers in the UK, students in the intervention showed greater improvements in self-esteem, as measured by the Rosenberg Self-Esteem Scale, and greater reductions in anxiety and depression, as measured by the Revised Children's Anxiety and Depression Scale-Short Version, at a 2-month follow-up compared to participants in a no-treatment control group (Perkins et al., 2021). A more recent example is *Project SOLVE*, a digital, self-guided intervention that teaches students about problem-solving in one 30-min session. In a trial with 357 middle schoolers in the USA, students in the intervention showed greater reductions in internalizing symptoms, as measured by the Behavior and Feelings Survey (Internalizing Subscale), at a 3-month follow-up compared to participants in an attention-matched control condition (Fitzpatrick et al., 2023).

Student-facing SSIs may also target mental health literacy, help-seeking intentions, or stigma. Recent systematic reviews show that several studies have investigated such SSIs (Hayes et al., 2023; Ma et al., 2023; Marinucci et al., 2023). For example, *Ending The Silence* is a 45-min SSI in which individuals with lived experience with mental illness give psychoeducational presentations to classes. In a trial with 232 high school students in New York, students who participated in the intervention had greater reductions in stigma, as measured by The Attitudes About Mental Illness and Its Treatment Scale, at the 4-week follow-up compared to students in an attention-matched control condition. Additionally, they had greater improvements in mental health knowledge, as measured by The Mental Health Knowledge Schedule, at the 8-week follow-up (DeLuca et al., 2021).

Teacher-, nurse-, or administrator-directed SSIs may be useful for promoting psychoeducation, which can in turn lead to a higher likelihood of identifying students with mental health concerns (Kidger et al., 2012; Whitley et al., 2013). Systematic reviews show that several educator-directed SSIs promoting mental health knowledge exist (Anderson et al., 2019; Yamaguchi et al., 2020). A recent example is *At-Risk for High School Educators*, a 45–60-min web-based intervention that includes role-play simulations with virtual humans to teach educators how to identify a student in distress, talk to that student, and make referrals to support services if necessary. In a trial with 31,144 high school educators across the USA, teachers who completed the intervention had greater improvements in preparedness, likelihood, and self-efficacy to engage in helping behaviors, as measured by the Gatekeeper Behavior Scale, at post-intervention compared to a waitlist control group (Albright et al., 2022).

Educator-directed SSIs could also instruct school personnel on how to help children with mental health conditions develop coping skills. For example, a freely available online SSI that teaches caregivers how to reduce anxiety in young children by reducing accommodation behaviors has proven effective and acceptable (Sung et al., 2021). Though the SSI was created for parents, educators could easily extrapolate the content to their roles. In addition to school staff, other individuals who interact with youth in the school system, such as mentors or paraprofessionals, could similarly benefit from these types of SSIs (Hart et al., 2023).

Given that burnout among school staff is an increasingly prevalent concern, staff-directed SSIs could be designed to target their own wellbeing or promote resilience (Pressley, 2021; Saloviita & Pakarinen, 2021). Later in this chapter, a case example is discussed that demonstrates the promise of SSIs for teacher wellbeing.

7.3.2   Multitiered Systems of Support

The target audience of school-based SSIs can also be described through a public health, multitiered systems lens. SSIs are well suited to be Tier 1 or Tier 2 supports. As described in Chap. 2, this volume, universal prevention programs, or Tier 1 programs, are those that target all students and/or personnel in a school setting, without selection based on current symptomatology or wellbeing (Gordon, 1983). Universal prevention programs aim to provide broadly applicable support tools for transdiagnostic mental health concerns, facilitate general psychoeducation, and determine which individuals may be in need of further intervention. Accessibility is integral to the successful implementation of universal prevention programs. Correspondingly, universal prevention programs should be minimally resource-intensive and easily implementable—two strengths of school-based SSIs.

One method for leveraging SSIs as universal prevention efforts is to include digital SSIs as part of the health curriculum, for example during a class period in a computer lab or as assigned homework. If time permits, instructors may facilitate conversations about the course content. However, many SSIs are designed to be self-administered. A dual purpose of these SSIs could be to determine which students may be in need of more intensive intervention. Students' responsiveness to SSIs, determined by changes in pre-post scores of psychological distress, may inform school personnel on whether to triage students to more robust supports. Similarly, it may be beneficial to require all teachers or other key staff to complete a psychoeducational SSI prior to the start of the school year to prepare for incoming students.

Tier 2 supports are more targeted programs that serve students who have been identified as being at-risk for mental health disorders or displaying subclinical levels of distress, and thus do not yet require intensive services. Such early identification and intervention before symptoms become impairing is imperative as such mild symptoms are often overlooked when they negatively affect academic achievement, socioemotional functioning, and serve as risk factors for poor outcomes in adulthood (Rutter et al., 2006). Tier 2 supports add to the efforts to prevent mental health disorders, effectively saving resources in the long term.

While more narrowly focused than Tier 1 supports, Tier 2 supports still aim to serve a large student population; thus, interventions need to be resource-efficient and scalable. Typically delivered in smaller, short-term group therapy sessions or via brief interventions administered at an individual level (e.g., daily teacher check-ins), SSIs are well positioned to step into this role. Digital, self-guided SSIs are readily available without wait times and can target a variety of problem areas (e.g., anxiety, attention, and organizational skills), as opposed to a "one-size fits all" approach of most Tier 2 supports, at the same time. Students who show declining symptoms in universal screening may be contacted by a school counselor or psychologist and be directed to an existing suite of school-supported SSIs. Students struggling with similar issues can also be grouped to complete the SSI together as well as benefit from peer support.

Given that SSIs do not require ongoing case management, schools may consider allocating resources to offering one-to-one SSI sessions in which a school counselor or psychologist helps select an appropriate SSI or if resources permit, walk the student through the SSI. Schools may also consider the implementation of single session consultation (SSC; https://osf.io/xnz2t/), a type of SSI that focuses on creating a goal-oriented action plan to address a specific, primary problem in the present moment or immediate future. The SSC is designed to be delivered by lay providers (e.g., teachers, school nurses, or counselors) and requires minimal training and ongoing supervision.

7.4   Case Example: WISE

The application of SSIs to educators has potential for widespread impact, both directly for adults and indirectly for students. It is widely known that education is a highly demanding profession that comes with many challenges. Teachers are historically overworked and underpaid, and they shoulder high levels of responsibility in an environment that offers little control (Gonzalez et al., 2008). In addition to facilitating academic performance, teachers are faced with supporting the growing mental health challenges of their students and maintaining a functional classroom, for which they receive little training (Ball et al., 2016). The unfortunate result is high levels of burnout and poor teacher retention, most prominently in communities that are historically marginalized. Nearly a third of teachers leave the profession within their first 5 years (Greenberg et al., 2016), a trend that has only been exacerbated by the COVID pandemic (Diliberti et al., 2021).

The impact of educator stress and turnover is felt widely. Teachers themselves are at a higher risk for mental health issues than most other professions (Schonfeld et al., 2017). In addition, educators hold the keys to student success by setting the culture and tone of a classroom, modeling effective regulation and interpersonal skills, being responsive and attuned to student needs, and ensuring that students feel safe, seen, and heard so their neurobiology is ripe for learning. Research has shown that teachers who are stressed have higher rates of classroom behavior problems, and depression in teachers is linked to poorer relational and academic outcomes for students (Hoglund, Klingle & Hosan, 2015; McLean & McDonald Connor, 2015; Roberts et al., 2016). And finally, educator retention issues can destabilize communities and exacerbate mental health and educational disparities that exist in under-resourced schools (Beteille et al., 2012).

Unfortunately, resources for addressing educator mental health and wellbeing are limited. Educators experience barriers to accessing traditional models of community care due to schedule limitations, stigma, and insurance restrictions. While embedded models of school-mental health are on the rise, the majority if not all of those resources go directly to students. Discouragingly, the current interventions that do exist for schools and educators tend to be time-consuming and less accessible, making educators an optimal target group for SSIs.

The Single Session Consultation (SSC) program is an SSI designed to provide solutions-focused support in a single, structured 30–90-min consultation session. SSC can be implemented by both clinicians and lay persons and was designed with scalability and system-level dissemination in mind. SSC has shown to be associated with increased hope and agency and decreased psychological distress in treatment-seeking individuals and is an effective strategy for supporting individuals wait-listed for ongoing psychotherapy (Schleider et al., 2021).

In an effort to gauge the utility and acceptability of SSC in the school setting, the MedStar Georgetown Center for Wellbeing in School Environments (WISE) began two new initiatives. First, WISE mental health clinicians were trained in SSC, and this service was added to WISE's Educator Therapy Program as an alternative intervention to care. The primary goal with this initiative was to increase access to care for those whom long-term psychotherapy was not a feasible or necessary path, as well as to manage waitlists for psychotherapy. Additionally, WISE began a pilot program for school leaders to receive training in SSC. This ongoing initiative aspires to build capacity for expanded mental health supports and sustainable, wall-to-wall cultures of wellbeing within schools.

For the clinician-focused initiative, WISE clinicians have found SSC to be an easily accessible intervention to learn and integrate into their clinical toolboxes. Clinicians also consistently report that SSC is an effective tool for diversifying clinical offerings to increase access to care and to reserve long-term psychotherapy services for individuals with the highest needs. Over 50 school personnel received SSC during the first year of implementation. Meaningful outcome data for this initiative are forthcoming. An initial attempt at program evaluation yielded eight individuals who endorsed receiving "short-term consultation" from WISE clinicians. While all participants noted some personal or professional benefit through open-ended questioning, findings are limited due to small sample size and inability to confirm that SSC was the modality used for those consultations.

For the capacity-building initiative, WISE held two trainings over a 3-month period. Participants were recruited via emails and flyers sent to partner schools. These communications described the intervention and sought to enlist any school personnel (including administrators, mental health professionals, and teachers) who self-identified as "a leader" within their schools and were interested in supporting the mental wellbeing of educators.

Training involved both asynchronous, individual pre-work and a synchronous, virtual group meeting. Participants first engaged in 90 min of asynchronous training materials from the Lab for Scalable Mental Health at Stony Brook University to provide a foundational understanding of SSC. Subsequently, a 2-h synchronous training was conducted by a WISE clinician and allowed participants to reflect on and answer questions about the asynchronous materials, receive instruction on therapeutic "soft skills" (e.g., mindset, body language, reflective listening), brainstorm and discuss logistics of implementation within schools, and watch skills be modeled. After the synchronous training, participants were paired up and instructed to engage in a "mock SSC session" with their partner before attempting to implement it within their schools.

At the end of the synchronous training, participants were asked to complete the Usage Rating Profile (URP-IR; Briesch et al., 2013) to assess perceived utility and feasibility of the intervention. The URP-IR utilizes a 6-point Likert scale with higher scores indicating greater endorsement. Subscales tap how well understood the intervention is (Understanding), how acceptable (Acceptability) and feasible (Feasibility) the intervention is perceived to be, and how much practical (System Support) and philosophical (System Climate) alignment are needed to implement the intervention (Briesch et al., 2013). Eleven participants across two training sessions completed the post-training survey. Findings indicated high levels of Acceptability ($M = 5.21$), Understanding ($M = 4.70$), Feasibility ($M = 4.83$), and System Climate ($M = 4.91$); and moderate levels of System Support needed ($M = 3.82$).

A follow-up survey was emailed to all participants 6–8 months after the synchronous training to assess for SSC implementation and barriers. Of the five respondents, three had implemented SSC in their schools, and all three rated the intervention as "somewhat" or "very" helpful. Three of the five participants also noted that the primary obstacle to implementation was "lack of opportunity to use SSC." Additional written responses suggested that most participants had not yet coordinated a whole school roll out, leading them to have to look for opportunities to utilize the skills less formally. In particular, teachers trained in SSC felt less comfortable applying the intervention informally in conversations with colleagues.

Overall, these initial pilot projects show promise for SSC as an efficient, accessible school-based intervention to enhance educator wellbeing. SSC can be easily adopted by mental health professionals who serve educators, allowing them to increase efficiency, expand reach, decrease barriers to engagement, and effectively manage waitlists. Additionally, there is interest in scaling SSC within schools and utilizing non-clinicians as SSC providers. In response to a growing number of requests, WISE is already slated to conduct four additional SSC trainings this year with school personnel. While more research is needed to understand the full impact and potential of SSC in schools, initial data show that school personnel find the SSC model to be acceptable, feasible, and understandable, especially after receiving enhanced training and support. SSC was also found to be helpful for those who implement it, but utilization within schools could be maximized through a whole-school approach where the intervention is advertised widely, the roles of SSC providers are clarified, and procedures exist for proactively and confidentially self-selecting into SSC.

7.5 Future Directions

7.5.1 Research

Implementation research is necessary to determine how school-based SSIs can fit into and enhance existing systems of support. For example, researchers should examine perceptions from students, teachers, school administrators, and other stakeholders regarding the barriers and facilitators of student-directed and/or educator-directed SSIs. Perceptions regarding in-person versus web-based SSIs additionally need to be understood. It is critical to assess what structural supports are needed to optimize uptake and awareness of SSIs among students and staff.

There are several other potential avenues for future research on school-based SSIs: (1) Given the goal of SSIs to alleviate overburdened systems of care, future research may examine long-term outcomes regarding the utilization of Tier 3 intensive treatments or crisis services after SSIs are embedded as Tier 1 or Tier 2 supports. It is possible that greater knowledge of mental health may lead to greater willingness to utilize intensive services. It is also possible that early prevention and skill building can lead to reduced need for intensive services. Future research may illuminate whether and in which circumstances SSIs contribute to changes in Tier 3 service utilization. (2) Given the detrimental effects that mental health concerns have on academic outcomes (Murphy et al., 2015), it is possible that student-directed SSIs targeting mental health outcomes may secondarily improve academic outcomes among students with high levels of distress, though evidence is needed to support this hypothesis. (3) Given the connection between teacher wellbeing and student wellbeing (Harding et al., 2019), it is possible that teacher-directed SSIs targeting their wellbeing may secondarily improve student wellbeing, yet this has not been tested. (4) Several SSIs have been designed to target mental health literacy, help-seeking intentions, or stigma among students, yet the majority of these interventions are delivered by trained facilitators or school staff. Additional research on self-administered SSIs to target mental health literacy, help-seeking intentions, or stigma is needed. (5) Existing school-based SSIs are largely static and untailored to students' specific needs (i.e., the content is the same for each student). Interventions that promote youth autonomy by giving them choices regarding which content or activities they are interested in, or interventions that adapt to students' unique needs by presenting content or activities according to students' self-identified symptoms or concerns, could improve outcomes and/or acceptability.

7.5.2 Policy Considerations

Implementing SSIs have many benefits to providing accessible and much needed mental health support to students. However, systematic structures or policies that support schools to realize the promise of SSIs are lacking. The need to increase funding at state and local levels to help schools promote mental health training for school staff, implement universal screening practices, and expand the workforce to provide mental health services (e.g., counselors, psychologists, social workers) has long been emphasized. However, Hoagwood et al. (2018) reported that research funding for children and adolescents' mental health services has decreased 42% from 2005 to 2015. Such a decrease in research funding is in direct contrast to the national priority to strengthen the mental health system capacity. While SSIs are resource-efficient, schools are a low-resourced and stretched setting, making it difficult for the uptake and maintenance of any added evidence-based services. Despite the plethora of evidence for the benefits of early identification and intervention of mental health problems and the promise the school settings offer, empirical evidence currently has failed to inform the important policy decisions around resource allocation and dissemination of effective interventions (Innvaer et al., 2002; Bogenschneider & Corbett, 2010).

Evidence-based policymaking is defined as "the systematic use of findings from program evaluations and outcome analyses ('evidence') to guide government policy and funding decisions" (Pew-MacArthur Results First Initiative, 2017, p. 4). However, research has found that policymakers are most reliant on personal contact, summaries with policy recommendations, and timely information when making policy decisions (Innvaer et al., 2002). Legislators reported that what they considered most important when looking at behavioral health research would be (1) data on budget impact, (2) cost-effectiveness analysis, and (3) brevity of the report (Purtle et al., 2018). Thus, it is critical for future research to consider the inclusion of economic evaluations as well as publishing brief reports that highlight their findings to successfully translate research for the public and its policymakers. It is clear that policy and clinical scientists share the goal of delivering mental health services to the biggest number of people possible while minimizing the costs of delivery and that the clinical science-to-policy gap can be bridged by increasing the shared common language between the two worlds.

7.6   Conclusion

To address the youth mental health crisis, innovative approaches for preventing and treating mental health problems are necessary. School-based SSIs offer one potential method for reaching youth in need of support who may otherwise be completely untreated and providing them with knowledge and skills that can alleviate distress. Among school personnel, SSIs can be used to increase knowledge of mental health and improve wellbeing, which may secondarily benefit students' mental health. The brief format of SSIs allows them to be easily integrated into existing school ecosystems as Tier 1 or Tier 2 services, which may serve to address students' needs before concerns are elevated to crises requiring intensive treatments. Further research is needed to understand how SSIs can be sustainably implemented in schools. Additionally, future research may investigate long-term outcomes such as utilization of crisis services and cost-effectiveness to evaluate the promise of SSIs to alleviate overburdened systems of care.

References

Albright, G., Fazel, M., Khalid, N., McMillan, J., Hilty, D., Shockley, K., & Joshi, S. (2022). High school educator training by simulation to address emotional and behavioral concerns in school settings: A randomized study. *Journal of Technology in Behavioral Science, 7*(3), 277–289. https://doi.org/10.1007/s41347-022-00243-9

Anderson, M., Werner-Seidler, A., King, C., Gayed, A., Harvey, S. B., & O'Dea, B. (2019). Mental health training programs for secondary school teachers: A systematic review. *School Mental Health, 11*(3), 489–508. https://doi.org/10.1007/s12310-018-9291-2

Baker, E. A., Brewer, S. K., Owens, J. S., Cook, C. R., & Lyon, A. R. (2021). Dissemination science in school mental health: A framework for future research. *School Mental Health, 13*(4), 791–807. https://doi.org/10.1007/s12310-021-09446-6

Ball, A., Iachini, A., Bohnenkamp, J., et al. (2016). School mental health content in state in-service K-12 teaching standards in the United States. *Teaching and Teacher Education, 60*, 312–320. https://doi.org/10.1016/j.tate.2016.08.020

Barkus, E., & Badcock, J. C. (2019). A transdiagnostic perspective on social anhedonia. *Frontiers in Psychiatry, 10*, 216. https://doi.org/10.3389/fpsyt.2019.00216

Béteille, T., Kalogrides, D., & Loeb, S. (2012). Stepping stones: Principal career paths and school outcomes. *Social Science Research, 41*(4), 904–919.

Bogenschneider, K., & Corbett, T. J. (2010). *Evidence-based policymaking: Insights from policy-minded researchers and research-minded policymakers.* Taylor & Francis.

Briesch, A. M., Chafouleas, S. M., Neugebauer, S. R., & Riley-Tillman, T. C. (2013). Assessing influences on intervention use: Revision of the usage rating profile-intervention. *Journal of School Psychology, 51*, 81–96. https://doi.org/10.1016/j.jsp.2012.08.006

Castellanos-Ryan, N., Brière, F. N., O'Leary-Barrett, M., Banaschewski, T., Bokde, A., Bromberg, U., Büchel, C., Flor, H., Frouin, V., Gallinat, J., Garavan, H., Martinot, J.-L., Nees, F., Paus, T., Pausova, Z., Rietschel, M., Smolka, M. N., Robbins, T. W., Whelan, R., et al. (2016). The structure of psychopathology in adolescence and its common personality and cognitive correlates. *Journal of Abnormal Psychology, 125*(8), 1039–1052. https://doi.org/10.1037/abn0000193

Cohen, K. A., Ito, S., Ahuvia, I. L., Yang, Y., Zhang, Y., Renshaw, T. L., Larson, M., Cook, C., Hill, S., Liao, J., Rapoport, A., Smock, A., Yang, M., & Schleider, J. L. (2024). Brief School-Based Interventions Targeting Student Mental Health or Well-Being: A Systematic Review and Meta-Analysis. *Clinical Child and Family Psychology Review.* https://doi.org/10.1007/s10567-024-00487-2

DeLuca, J. S., Tang, J., Zoubaa, S., Dial, B., & Yanos, P. T. (2021). Reducing stigma in high school students: A cluster randomized controlled trial of the National Alliance on Mental Illness' Ending the Silence intervention. *Stigma and Health, 6*(2), 228–242. https://doi.org/10.1037/sah0000235

Diliberti, M. K., Schwartz, H. L., & Grant, D. M. (2021). *Stress topped the reasons why public school teachers quit, even before COVID-19.* RAND.

Dimitropoulos, G., Cullen, J., Cullen, O., Pawluk, C., McLuckie, A., Patten, S., Bulloch, A., Wilcox, G., & Arnold, P. D. (2022). "Teachers often see the red flags first": Perceptions of school staff regarding their roles in supporting students with mental health concerns. *School Mental Health, 14*(2), 402–415. https://doi.org/10.1007/s12310-021-09475-1

Dobias, M. L., Schleider, J. L., Jans, L., & Fox, K. R. (2021). An online, single-session intervention for adolescent self-injurious thoughts and behaviors: Results from a randomized trial. *Behaviour Research and Therapy, 147*, 103983. https://doi.org/10.1016/j.brat.2021.103983

Duong, M. T., Bruns, E. J., Lee, K., Cox, S., Coifman, J., Mayworm, A., & Lyon, A. R. (2021). Rates of mental health service utilization by children and adolescents in schools and other common service settings: A systematic review and meta-analysis. *Administration and Policy in Mental Health, 48*(3), 420–439. https://doi.org/10.1007/s10488-020-01080-9

Eccles, A. M., Qualter, P., Madsen, K. R., & Holstein, B. E. (2020). Loneliness in the lives of Danish adolescents: Associations with health and sleep. *Scandinavian Journal of Public Health, 48*(8), 877–887. https://doi.org/10.1177/1403494819865429

Fazel, M., Hoagwood, K., Stephan, S., & Ford, T. (2014). Mental health interventions in schools in high-income countries. *The Lancet Psychiatry, 1*(5), 377–387. https://doi.org/10.1016/S2215-0366(14)70312-8

Fitzpatrick, O. M., Schleider, J. L., Mair, P., Carson, A., Harisinghani, A., & Weisz, J. R. (2023). Project SOLVE: Randomized, school-based trial of a single-session digital problem-solving intervention for adolescent internalizing symptoms during the coronavirus era. *School Mental Health, 15*, 955. https://doi.org/10.1007/s12310-023-09598-7

Gonzalez, L., Brown, M. S., & Slate, J. R. (2008). Teachers who left the teaching profession: A qualitative understanding. *The Qualitative Report, 13*(1), 1–11. https://doi.org/10.46743/2160-3715/2008.1601

Gordon, R. S. (1983). An operational classification of disease prevention. *Public Health Reports, 98*(2), 107–109.

Greenberg, M., Brown, J., & Abenavoli, R. (2016). *Teacher stress and health: Effects on teachers, students, and schools*. Pennsylvania State University.

Gruber, J., Prinstein, M. J., Clark, L. A., Rottenberg, J., Abramowitz, J. S., Albano, A. M., Aldao, A., Borelli, J. L., Chung, T., Davila, J., Forbes, E. E., Gee, D. G., Hall, G. C. N., Hallion, L. S., Hinshaw, S. P., Hofmann, S. G., Hollon, S. D., Joormann, J., Kazdin, A. E., et al. (2021). Mental health and clinical psychological science in the time of COVID-19: Challenges, opportunities, and a call to action. *American Psychologist, 76*(3), 409–426. https://doi.org/10.1037/amp0000707

Harding, S., Morris, R., Gunnell, D., Ford, T., Hollingworth, W., Tilling, K., Evans, R., Bell, S., Grey, J., Brockman, R., Campbell, R., Araya, R., Murphy, S., & Kidger, J. (2019). Is teachers' mental health and wellbeing associated with students' mental health and wellbeing? *Journal of Affective Disorders, 242*, 180–187. https://doi.org/10.1016/j.jad.2018.08.080

Hart, M. J., Sable, R., Gupta, A., Boddu, J., & McQuillin, S. D. (2022). Adapting a school-based motivational interviewing mentoring program for use in India. *School Psychology International, 43*(2), 196–216. https://doi.org/10.1177/01430343221080782

Hart, M. J., Sung, J. Y., McQuillin, S. D., & Schleider, J. L. (2023). Expanding the reach of psychosocial services for youth: Untapped potential of mentor-delivered single session interventions. *Journal of Community Psychology, 51*(3), 1255–1272. https://doi.org/10.1002/jcop.22927

Hayes, D., Mansfield, R., Mason, C., Santos, J., Moore, A., Boehnke, J., Ashworth, E., Moltrecht, B., Humphrey, N., Stallard, P., Patalay, P., & Deighton, J. (2023). The impact of universal, school based, interventions on help seeking in children and young people: A systematic literature review. *European Child & Adolescent Psychiatry*. https://doi.org/10.1007/s00787-022-02135-y

Herrenkohl, T. I. (2019). Cross-system collaboration and engagement of the public health model to promote the well-being of children and families. *Journal of the Society for Social Work and Research, 10*(3), 319–332. https://doi.org/10.1086/704958

Hoagwood, K. E., Atkins, M., Kelleher, K., Peth-Pierce, R., Olin, S., Burns, B., Landsverk, J., & Horwitz, S. M. (2018). Trends in children's mental health services research funding by the National Institute of Mental Health from 2005 to 2015: A 42% reduction. *Journal of the American Academy of Child and Adolescent Psychiatry, 57*(1), 10–13. https://doi.org/10.1016/j.jaac.2017.09.433

Hoglund, W. L., Klingle, K. E., & Hosan, N. E. (2015). Classroom risks and resources: Teacher burnout, classroom quality and children's adjustment in high needs elementary schools. *Journal of School Psychology, 53*(5), 337–357.

Innvær, S., Vist, G., Trommald, M., & Oxman, A. (2002). Health policy-makers' perceptions of their use of evidence: A systematic review. *Journal of Health Services Research & Policy, 7*(4), 239–244. https://doi.org/10.1258/135581902320432778

Kazdin, A. E. (2017). Addressing the treatment gap: A key challenge for extending evidence-based psychosocial interventions. *Behaviour Research and Therapy, 88*, 7–18. https://doi.org/10.1016/j.brat.2016.06.004

Kazdin, A. E. (2019). Annual research review: Expanding mental health services through novel models of intervention delivery. *Journal of Child Psychology and Psychiatry, and Allied Disciplines, 60*(4), 455–472. https://doi.org/10.1111/jcpp.12937

Kidger, J., Araya, R., Donovan, J., & Gunnell, D. (2012). The effect of the school environment on the emotional health of adolescents: A systematic review. *Pediatrics, 129*(5), 925–949. https://doi.org/10.1542/peds.2011-2248

Love, H. E., Schlitt, J., Soleimanpour, S., Panchal, N., & Behr, C. (2019). Twenty years of school-based health care growth and expansion. *Health Affairs, 38*(5), 755–764. https://doi.org/10.1377/hlthaff.2018.05472

Lyon, A. (2021). Designing programs with an eye toward scaling. In J. List, D. Suskind, & L. Supplee (Eds.), *The scale-up effect in early childhood & public policy: Why interventions lose impact at scale and what we can do about it*. Routledge.

Ma, K. K. Y., Anderson, J. K., & Burn, A.-M. (2023). Review: School-based interventions to improve mental health literacy and reduce mental health stigma – A systematic review. *Child and Adolescent Mental Health, 28*(2), 230–240. https://doi.org/10.1111/camh.12543

Marinucci, A., Grové, C., & Allen, K.-A. (2023). A scoping review and analysis of mental health literacy interventions for children and youth. *School Psychology Review, 52*(2), 144–158. https://doi.org/10.1080/2372966X.2021.2018918

McDanal, R., Parisi, D., Opara, I., & Schleider, J. L. (2022). Effects of brief interventions on internalizing symptoms and substance use in youth: A systematic review. *Clinical Child and Family Psychology Review, 25*(2), 339–355. https://doi.org/10.1007/s10567-021-00372-2

McLean, L., & Connor, C. M. (2015). Depressive symptoms in third-grade teachers: Relations to classroom quality and student achievement. *Child Development, 86*(3), 945–954.

Murphy, J. M., Guzmán, J., McCarthy, A., Squicciarini, A. M., George, M., Canenguez, K., Dunn, E. C., Baer, L., Simonsohn, A., Smoller, J. W., & Jellinek, M. (2015). Mental health predicts better academic outcomes: A longitudinal study of elementary school students in Chile. *Child Psychiatry and Human Development, 46*(2), 245–256. https://doi.org/10.1007/s10578-014-0464-4

Organisation for Economic Cooperation and Development. (2020). *Curriculum overload: A way forward*. OECD Publishing. https://doi.org/10.1787/3081ceca-en

Ormiston, H. E., Nygaard, M. A., & Apgar, S. (2022). A systematic review of secondary traumatic stress and compassion fatigue in teachers. *School Mental Health, 14*(4), 802–817. https://doi.org/10.1007/s12310-022-09525-2

Osborn, T. L., Rodriguez, M., Wasil, A. R., Venturo-Conerly, K. E., Gan, J., Alemu, R. G., Roe, E., Arango, G. S., Otieno, B. H., Wasanga, C. M., Shingleton, R., & Weisz, J. R. (2020). Single-session digital intervention for adolescent depression, anxiety, and well-being: Outcomes of a randomized controlled trial with Kenyan adolescents. *Journal of Consulting and Clinical Psychology, 88*(7), 657–668. https://doi.org/10.1037/ccp0000505

Öst, L.-G., & Ollendick, T. H. (2017). Brief, intensive and concentrated cognitive behavioral treatments for anxiety disorders in children: A systematic review and meta-analysis. *Behaviour Research and Therapy, 97*, 134–145. https://doi.org/10.1016/j.brat.2017.07.008

Panchal, N., Cox, C., & Rudowitz, R. (2022). *The landscape of school-based mental health services*. Kaiser Family Foundation.

Perkins, A. M., Bowers, G., Cassidy, J., Meiser-Stedman, R., & Pass, L. (2021). An enhanced psychological mindset intervention to promote adolescent wellbeing within educational settings: A feasibility randomized controlled trial. *Journal of Clinical Psychology, 77*(4), 946–967. https://doi.org/10.1002/jclp.23104

Pressley, T. (2021). Factors contributing to teacher burnout during COVID-19. *Educational Researcher, 50*(5), 325–327. https://doi.org/10.3102/0013189X211004138

Purtle, J., Dodson, E. A., Nelson, K., Meisel, Z. F., & Brownson, R. C. (2018). Legislators' sources of behavioral Health Research and preferences for dissemination: Variations by political party. *Psychiatric Services, 69*(10), 1105–1108.

Radez, J., Reardon, T., Creswell, C., Orchard, F., & Waite, P. (2022). Adolescents' perceived barriers and facilitators to seeking and accessing professional help for anxiety and depressive disorders: A qualitative interview study. *European Child & Adolescent Psychiatry, 31*(6), 891–907. https://doi.org/10.1007/s00787-020-01707-0

Roberts, A., LoCasale-Crouch, J., Hamre, B., & DeCoster, J. (2016). Exploring teachers' depressive symptoms, interaction quality, and children's social-emotional development in Head Start. *Early Education and Development, 27*(5), 642–654.

Robinson, L. E., Valido, A., Drescher, A., Woolweaver, A. B., Espelage, D. L., LoMurray, S., Long, A. C. J., Wright, A. A., & Dailey, M. M. (2023). Teachers, stress, and the COVID-19 pandemic: A qualitative analysis. *School Mental Health, 15*(1), 78–89. https://doi.org/10.1007/s12310-022-09533-2

Rutter, M., Kim-Cohen, J., & Maughan, B. (2006). Continuities and discontinuities in psychopathology between childhood and adult life. *Journal of Child Psychology and Psychiatry, and Allied Disciplines, 47*(3–4), 276–295. https://doi.org/10.1111/j.1469-7610.2006.01614.x

Saloviita, T., & Pakarinen, E. (2021). Teacher burnout explained: Teacher-, student-, and organisation-level variables. *Teaching and Teacher Education, 97*, 103221. https://doi.org/10.1016/j.tate.2020.103221

Schleider, J. L., & Weisz, J. R. (2017). Little treatments, promising effects? Meta-analysis of single-session interventions for youth psychiatric problems. *Journal of the American Academy of Child and Adolescent Psychiatry, 56*(2), 107–115. https://doi.org/10.1016/j.jaac.2016.11.007

Schleider, J. L., & Weisz, J. (2018). A single-session growth mindset intervention for adolescent anxiety and depression: 9-month outcomes of a randomized trial. *Journal of Child Psychology and Psychiatry, and Allied Disciplines, 59*(2), 160–170. https://doi.org/10.1111/jcpp.12811

Schleider, J. L., Dobias, M. L., Sung, J. Y., & Mullarkey, M. C. (2020a). Future directions in single-session youth mental health interventions. *Journal of Clinical Child and Adolescent Psychology, 49*(2), 264–278. https://doi.org/10.1080/15374416.2019.1683852

Schleider, J. L., Dobias, M., Sung, J., Mumper, E., & Mullarkey, M. (2020b). Acceptability and utility of an open-access, online single-session intervention platform for adolescent mental health. *JMIR Mental Health, 7*(6), e20513. https://doi.org/10.2196/20513

Schleider, J. L., Sung, J., Bianco, A., Gonzalez, A., Vivian, D., & Mullarkey, M. C. (2021). Open pilot trial of a single-session consultation service for clients on psychotherapy wait-lists. In *The behavior therapist* (Vol. 44, pp. 8–15). https://doi.org/10.31234/osf.io/fdwqk

Schonfeld, I. S., Bianchi, R., & Luehring-Jones, P. (2017). Consequences of job stress for the mental health of teachers. In T. McIntyre, S. McIntyre, & D. Francis (Eds.), *Educator stress (Aligning perspectives on health, safety and well-being).* Springer. https://doi.org/10.1007/978-3-319-53053-6_3

Shen, J., Rubin, A., Cohen, K., Hart, E. A., Sung, J., McDanal, R., Roulston, C., Sotomayor, I., Fox, K. R., & Schleider, J. L. (2023). Randomized evaluation of an online single-session intervention for minority stress in LGBTQ+ adolescents. *Internet Interventions, 33*, 100633. https://doi.org/10.1016/j.invent.2023.100633

Sung, J. Y., Mumper, E., & Schleider, J. L. (2021). Empowering anxious parents to manage child avoidance behaviors: Randomized control trial of a single-session intervention for parental accommodation. *JMIR Mental Health, 8*(7), e29538. https://doi.org/10.2196/29538

Sung, J. Y., Bugatti, M., Vivian, D., & Schleider, J. L. (2023). Evaluating a telehealth single-session consultation service for clients on psychotherapy wait-lists. *Practice Innovations, 8*(2), 141–161. https://doi.org/10.1037/pri0000207

The Pew Charitable Trusts. (2017). *How states engage in evidence-based policymaking.* https://www.pewtrusts.org/en/research-and-analysis/reports/2017/01/how-states-engage-in-evidence-based-policymaking

Weisz, J. R., Kuppens, S., Ng, M. Y., Eckshtain, D., Ugueto, A. M., Vaughn-Coaxum, R., Jensen-Doss, A., Hawley, K. M., Krumholz Marchette, L. S., Chu, B. C., Weersing, V. R., & Fordwood, S. R. (2017). What five decades of research tells us about the effects of youth psychological therapy: A multilevel meta-analysis and implications for science and practice. *The American Psychologist, 72*(2), 79–117. https://doi.org/10.1037/a0040360

Whitley, J., Smith, J. D., & Vaillancourt, T. (2013). Promoting mental health literacy among educators: Critical in school-based prevention and intervention. *Canadian Journal of School Psychology, 28*(1), 56–70. https://doi.org/10.1177/0829573512468852

Yamaguchi, S., Foo, J. C., Nishida, A., Ogawa, S., Togo, F., & Sasaki, T. (2020). Mental health literacy programs for school teachers: A systematic review and narrative synthesis. *Early Intervention in Psychiatry, 14*(1), 14–25. https://doi.org/10.1111/eip.12793

Chapter 8
Reaching Traditionally Underserved Populations: School-Based Interventions to Create Safe and Welcoming Schools for Immigrant Students and Families

Germán A. Cadenas, Vanesa Luna, Lorena Tule-Romain, Viridiana Carrizales, Marsha Akoto, Cheryl Aguilar, Raquel Sosa, Vindhyaa Pasupuleti, and Emmanuel Ogunkoya

8.1 Reaching Traditionally Underserved Populations: School-Based Interventions to Create Safe and Welcoming Schools for Undocumented Students and Families

The demographics of the United States at large, as well as its Kindergarten through 12th grade schools (K-12), are changing rapidly, with growing diversity driving these changes. The U.S. Census Bureau (2019) estimated that about half of youth enrolled in K-12 schools in 2018 were youth of color, including Latinx (25% of

---

Note: We would like to thank Genesis Genao, undergraduate student at Lehigh University, for her support to the authors in gathering and reviewing literature for this chapter.

G. A. Cadenas (✉)
Graduate School of Applied & Professional Psychology, Rutgers University New Brunswick, Piscataway, NJ, USA
e-mail: german.cadenas@rutgers.edu

V. Luna
ImmSchools, Brooklyn, NY, USA
e-mail: vanessa@immschools.org

L. Tule-Romain
ImmSchools, Dallas, TX, USA
e-mail: lorena@immschools.org

V. Carrizales
ImmSchools, Bulverde, TX, USA
e-mail: viridiana@immschools.org

© The Author(s), under exclusive license to Springer Nature Switzerland AG 2024
L. Kern et al. (eds.), *Scaling Effective School Mental Health Interventions and Practices*,
https://doi.org/10.1007/978-3-031-68168-4_8

youth in K-12 schools), Black (15%), and Asian (5%). These communities are experiencing the most growth among its youth, yet these are also racially and ethnically minoritized groups that have been historically underserved by educational practices and policies. Immigrant students also represent a significant portion of the students in K-12 schools. Approximately five million (or 10%) K-12 students in the United States are either undocumented or live in a mixed-status household (i.e., family with members who have varied immigration statuses from temporary to legal to no status), and one in four students is an immigrant or comes from an immigrant family (Zong & Batalova, 2019). Although schools are legally and morally obligated to protect and serve immigrant students, teachers and school leaders rarely have the resources and skills they need to live up to this obligation. This lack of competent preparedness leads to inequality in educational engagement, school mental health (SMH) programming, educational outcomes, and well-being of immigrant youth.

Immigrant youth and families experience unique stressors and needs (e.g., legal status barriers), which K-12 schools may not be fully prepared to address (Suárez-Orozco et al., 2015). This creates school environments where immigrant students do not feel included or safe. Attending schools that are not responsive to their needs may expose immigrant students to risks to their socioemotional development, educational success, pathways to college, and overall well-being (Gonzales, 2016; Gonzales & Chavez, 2012; Nienhusser, 2013). Additionally, school educators and SMH leaders may need specialized supports to develop competencies and create more welcoming schools, and these supports may vary greatly by state based on policies, funding, standards, and teacher training (Gonzales, 2010; Jefferies & Dabach, 2014). Hence, specialized multitiered interventions are needed to promote positive outcomes among immigrant youth and families, and to prepare school educators and SMH leaders and staff to better serve these youth and their families.

Extant research suggests key areas to focus multitier educational and SMH interventions in order to alleviate and reduce inequitable programming and resources for immigrant youth. Specifically, extant research supports (a) the relevance of empowering immigrant youth and families with resources that may lead to increases in school engagement and educational outcomes (Cadenas et al., 2021; Cisneros &

M. Akoto · R. Sosa
Department of Education and Human Services, Lehigh University, Bethlehem, PA, USA
e-mail: maa821@lehigh.edu; ras619@lehigh.edu

C. Aguilar
School for Social Work, Smith College, Northampton, MA, USA
e-mail: caguilar@thehopecenterforwellness.com

V. Pasupuleti
ImmSchools, New York, NY, USA
e-mail: vindhyaa@immschools.org

E. Ogunkoya
ImmSchools, Houston, TX, USA
e-mail: emmanuel@immschools.org

Cadenas, 2017; Crawford & Valle, 2016; Suárez-Orozco et al., 2009; Torres-Olave et al., 2021; Motti-Stefanidi & Masten, 2013) and (b) that it is key to partner with educators, administrators, and SMH leaders and staff to develop their cultural competencies to facilitate and advocate for the success of immigrant youth (Amuedo-Dorantes et al., 2022; Crawford & Dorner 2019; Todd et al., 2020; Parkhouse et al., 2020). Furthermore, conducting research with immigrant youth and families in a participatory manner is recommended as a next step to reduce the inequalities they experience and to ensure that findings and strategies that emanate from them accurately reflect the lived experiences, challenges, and assets of their communities (Suárez-Orozco et al., 2015). Importantly, interventions for supporting the psychological well-being of immigrant youth can be conceptualized as Tier 1 since they are oriented toward addressing the cultural, structural, and systemic factors within schools and districts (Arora et al., 2021; Cadenas et al., 2019; Marsh & Mathur, 2020). However, research exploring innovative educational and SMH strategies for immigrant youth and families is lacking (Suárez-Orozco et al., 2015). Addressing this need, this chapter provides a synthesis of the literature pertaining to the link between (a) school participation and SMH, and (b) culturally informed education and SMH programming for immigrant students and their families.

Furthermore, this chapter describes the Tier 1 intervention programs provided by Immschools, a nonprofit organization that partners with schools to provide specialized support programs to immigrant youth and families, educators, and school and SMH leaders and staff. These programs are designed to transform schools to become more inclusive and safer for immigrant students. Additionally, these programs are participatory, implemented with input, feedback, and guidance of a Community Advisory Board composed of current and former immigrant youth. In 2024, ImmSchools was providing services in K-12 public and private urban schools in New York (New York City), New Jersey (Camden), and Texas (Dallas Fort Worth and San Antonio). This chapter also describes the ImmSchools Participatory Action Research (PAR) Study, which aims to establish an evidence base for ImmSchools Tier 1 educational intervention programs, with the goal of sharing effective intervention components with the public and policymakers to encourage widespread adoption of these interventions to reduce inequitable educational and mental health outcomes for immigrant youth.

8.2 School Participation and School Mental Health

8.2.1 School Participation and Mental Health of Underserved Students and Families

The influence of schools on students' lives extends far beyond educational outcomes. School participation has been associated with improvement in the school environment, relationships, and positive health and well-being outcomes

(John-Akinola & Nic-Gabhainn, 2014). Despite this important connection, research points to several factors that are associated with decreased school involvement of immigrant families, such as socioeconomic status, structural barriers, and language barriers. For example, Crosnoe and Turley (2011) suggested that immigrant parents who experience language barriers engage in visible school-related involvement such as parent-school meetings with less frequency than parents of youth born in the United States. While it is important to consider barriers to school participation, it is also crucial to identify the other ways in which immigrant parents are involved in their children's educational goals outside of the school system, such as instilling positive values and hard work ethics (Crosnoe & Turley 2011).

8.2.2 School Participation and Mental Health of Undocumented Students and Families

Immigrant students and families face a myriad of stressors due to their immigration status that serve as barriers to learning, school participation, and socioemotional development. Critical steps toward supporting these students' well-being and enhance their school participation are to acknowledge the strengths held by immigrant students and families, an to recognize that immigration status is a social determinant of health (Cha et al., 2019). Although many immigrant students share similar challenges, there is variability in functioning of all school communities and diversity in experiences of immigrant students and their families (Hernandez et al., 2010). The way in which stressors impact immigrants and youth vary depending upon their developmental stages during migration; their coping mechanisms; the length of time in the country; the limitations and/or access to resources available to them and their families; familial supports available; structural barriers; experiences of racism and discrimination; the influence of local politics and community cultures; and the nature of pre-migration, during and after migration journeys (e.g., stressors and trauma experienced at country of origin, during migration journey, and/or in their new communities in the United States) (Gonzales et al., 2013, 2014). The links between immigration status and acculturative stress, worry about the future, stigma, hopelessness, and feelings of isolation have been well established in the literature (Kemmak et al., 2021). These stressors present as risk factors for mental health challenges among immigrants (Diaz & Fenning, 2021).

For instance, fear associated with exposure of immigration status may lead to isolation and withdrawal from networks and opportunities (Gonzales, et al., 2013). Further, students who live within mixed-status families (e.g., in relation to legal immigration status) may experience preoccupation about others and/or their own status and complexities when some family members have access to resources and opportunities based on their statuses and others do not (Fix & Zimmermann, 2001). These students may experience a sense of hopelessness when they become aware of their immigration statuses and miss important age-related milestones, such as obtaining a driver's license, voting, and obtaining after-school jobs (Gonzales et al., 2013). Research points to a phenomenon deemed the *immigrant paradox* attributed to a student's length of time in the United States. Length of time in the country has been found to be a protective factor for newly arrived immigrants (e.g., first-generation immigrants), while other studies have found a connection of length of time with declining academic achievement and aspirations (Suárez-Orozco et al., 2009). These mixed findings suggest that some immigrant youth may hold protective mechanisms that support their well-being when they arrive in the United States, while subsequent generations of immigrants may lose these advantages. Hence, an important implication is for schools to consider youths' immigrant generation in the United States when assessing for needs and developing appropriate SMH interventions. Another common concern for some students is fear of deportation, which has been associated with a negative impact on self-image (Cavazos-Rehg et al., 2007). For undocumented immigrants who have grown up in the United States and socialized in a school environment, shame and stigma regarding their immigration status, as well as an ongoing lack of belonging, have been associated with their greater mental health concerns, such as chronic stress, hopelessness, and disruptions in identity development (Abrego, 2011; Gonzales, et al., 2013). Hence, it is important that SMH providers assess for sense of belonging, shame, and stigma among immigrant youth, as well as the impact of the school climate.

While gaining English language skills may initially generate stress, frustration, and adversely impact social nuances and academic performance (Suárez-Orozco et al., 2009), when students gain English proficiency and acquire other skills, they also gain a sense of pride, capacity, and empowerment (Diaz & Fenning, 2021). With new skills, students may transition to serve as "cultural, social and political brokers" (Sigona et al., 2019, p. 134) to their parents and families, roles that can foster a sense of pride, helpfulness, and increased resilience (Diaz & Fenning, 2021). This entails youth fulfilling familial roles where they translate, interpret, educate, and advocate with and for their families to help them navigate and function in a new country, particularly within the education system. Children and youth who serve as their family's brokers are often identified in the literature as parentified children. While these students may appear as responsible, high-functioning helpers, they can experience feelings of isolation, low self-esteem, anxiety, and depression during childhood, and their own needs may go unnoticed (Cheng, 2012). Hence, it is important that SMH programming is provided across multiple tiers of intervention to meet mental health needs that may not be easily observable among immigrant youth. Furthermore, SMH providers and schools may intervene at the Tier 1 level to provide information and resources to parents directly (e.g., education about legal rights), and by doing so take the burden off the youth to find and make sense of information and resources alone.

In addition to immigration status as a stressor, immigrant youth and their families have consistently been affected by other social determinants of health such as low-economic status, food and housing insecurity, and challenges with health care access (Arora et al., 2021; Cadenas et al., 2022). A growing body of literature is making more explicit the systemic/structural conditions that negatively impact the mental health of immigrant communities (Kemmak et al., 2021). While challenges exist among immigrants, protective factors also exist among immigrant youth broadly and among undocumented students and their families specifically. Factors such as cultural values, religiosity, spirituality, ethnic identity (Garcini et al., 2021), resiliency, and ability to adapt (Lad & Braganza, 2013) have been found to play an important role in protecting and promoting positive mental health among these students and their communities.

8.3 Culturally Informed Educational Practices and School Mental Health

8.3.1 Culturally Informed Educational Practices

Culturally informed practices are rooted in multicultural education, which grew out of the Civil Rights movement in an attempt to bring structural and systemic changes in the US education systems (Banks, 1989; Davidman & Davidman, 1997). According to Gay (2004), multicultural education and culturally responsive approaches are described as sharing a *"common goal to teach contributions of cultural diverse groups and develop social consciousness, civic responsibility, and political activism to reconstruct society for greater pluralistic equality, truth, inclusion and justice"* (p. 32). Culturally informed educational practices are of necessary importance, as they provide many positive outcomes to students' learning, development, and performance, among others (Gay, 2010a, b). Alternatively, the lack of culturally informed education practices can lead to negative outcomes in students' academic performance and psychological well-being (Cholewa et al., 2014). Culturally informed practices impact educational systems on multiple levels, such as on policies at the school and district level, administrative processes, approaches to leadership, educational practices in the classroom, provision of SMH programs and services, and mentoring and advising of students. Each level of impact has implications on the way that diverse students, including immigrant youth, are supported, how they engage in education, and how this context is facilitative of positive mental health.

Past research suggests that a safe, welcoming, and culturally competent school environment can promote a sense of community, friendships, and belonging (Korpershoek et al., 2021). Implementing culturally informed practices is an approach to creating safe and welcoming spaces for immigrant youth, within which their emotional health may thrive. Moreover, culturally informed practices to support immigrant youth can be implemented through macro-level policies in schools, school hiring processes, school curricula, and micro-level work done in the classroom between educators and students. Researchers demonstrated that educational workshops and professional development programs that provide factual information about immigrant communities, tackle anti-immigrant biases held by educators, and center the lived experiences and narratives of young immigrants can serve to enhance the cultural responsiveness and competencies of educators to serve immigrant youth (Cisneros & Cadenas, 2017; Cadenas et al., 2018).

8.3.2 Anti-racism and Culturally Informed Education Practices

The US educational system has a long-standing history rooted in racism. From Separate but Equal segregation doctrine, to institutional barriers (e.g., exclusive learning environments, culturally incompetent practices among educators and school counselors, and poorly trained and understaffed educators), racism in the US education system is still very prevalent and impacts minoritized and immigrant students and their parents as they receive educational and SMH services that are not culturally affirming and unwelcoming of their cultural identities (Constantine & Gushue, 2003; Qin et al., 2022). Immigrant students are likely to attend schools that are segregated, resource deficient, and unwelcoming (Suárez-Orozco et al., 2009). This subsequently impacts student engagement in school and performance, creates educational disparities, and has perpetuated gaps in achievement between immigrant and youth who are born in the United States (Suárez-Orozco et al., 2015). Research suggests that racism and discrimination toward groups of immigrants impact the school environment by creating a sense of "otherness" toward these students, hence impeding their successful integration within schools and the larger community, and impeding outcomes related to mental health, physical health, and educational development (Metzner et al., 2022). Structural racism within school policies and practices is manifested in the form of culturally insensitive SMH that perpetuate mental health disparities.

There are many approaches that educators can take to promote psychological well-being and academic achievement among students of color. Past research has shown the efficacy of culturally informed and culturally responsive education practices in mitigating racism and creating an anti-racist education environment. Multicultural education is described as reform that school and other educational institutions implement in the hope that students of color, racially ethnic, and social-class groups will experience educational equality (Banks, 1993; p. 4 and p. 20). Approaches that educators can take to create a more inclusive and anti-racist environment include the following: (a) helping students develop racial attitudes (i.e., emotions, beliefs, and predispositions toward groups of people based on their race) by exploring their racial identity in relation to the context of racism and discrimination of minoritized groups, (b) implementing ethnic content into the school curriculum to help center the experiences of minoritized groups, and (c) educating children about the histories of different racial and ethnic groups that tend to be unaddressed in K-12 education curriculum (Banks, 2001). Hence, infusing anti-racism within the curriculum and other educational practices can be considered a Tier 1 type of intervention to reduce discrimination and thereby alleviate mental health concerns among students of color, including immigrants.

8.3.3 Culturally Informed Educational Practices for Undocumented Students

In the US K-12 education system, there are approximately 2.2 million immigrant children, including 100,000 undocumented students who graduate from high school every year (Capps et al., 2016; Zong & Batalova, 2019). Immigration has been found to increase children's risk of developing many challenges such as internalizing and externalizing problems (Chan 2001). Racist, anti-immigrant, and xenophobic rhetoric create unsafe and unwelcoming spaces for immigrant students, especially Latinx and Muslim students (Sidhu, 2017). Acculturative stress (e.g., stress related to immigrants navigating the culture and norms of the dominant group), immigration-related stress, language barriers, family separation, among other factors contribute to higher rates of poor mental health in immigrant students, and a lack of sense of belonging (Coll et al., 2012). Furthermore, immigrant and undocumented students face several challenges in their development, including segregation and exclusion in schools, lack of access to services that affirm multilingualism among youth and families, and educational practices that fail to engage youth and families from diverse countries of origin (Coll & Marks, 2012; Coll et al., 2012). Due to the increased risk of poor psychological well-being for immigrant students, it is important for educators to implement policies, practices, and interventions that create safe inclusive spaces of immigrant and undocumented students, where their sense of agency (e.g., perceived ability), ambition, initiative, and overall mental health may flourish (Bandura, 2006; Arora et al., 2021). However, there is sparse literature about specific interventions to support undocumented students. Section 8.3.5 offers specific recommendations to help guide educators and SMH service providers in working with this population.

8.3.4 Culturally Informed Practices and Educators' Mental Health

As evidenced by past research, teacher burnout is due but not limited to feelings of inadequacy, lack of support, and poor working conditions (Xie et al., 2022). As a result, schools are at increased risk for high turnover, as teacher's psychological well-being contributes significantly to the climate within the school (Xie et al., 2022; Grayson & Alvarez, 2008). Moreover, teachers' lack of multicultural competencies and culturally informed practices related to mental health subsequently influence the ability to support immigrant students. Scholars have posited that educators' perceptions of immigrant students as an asset, in contrast to viewing them as problematic, was related to lower diversity-related burnout and a greater sense of agency to support and serve as an educator for immigrant students (Grayson & Alvarez, 2008; Gutentag et al., 2018). In a similar vein, recent research has examined teacher practices in relation to educators' denial of seeing ideological or structural racism (i.e., color-blind racial attitudes), with findings illustrating that this form of racism is detrimental to educators' ability to develop agency in culturally informed practices to serve immigrants (Cadenas et al., 2021). Hence, a growing literature is documenting the links between culturally informed practices and educators' overall competence to work with immigrants (e.g., agency in their educational practices) and educators' overall well-being (e.g., burnout).

8.3.5 Interventions to Promote Culturally Informed Practices and Mental Health

Past research suggests that there are many approaches educators can take to implement culturally informed practices. Working closely with family members and students, creating heterogeneous curricula that are representative of diverse student populations, becoming competent in language acquisition theories to inform education practices with language learned, and participating in ongoing professional training are interventions that can help educators support immigrant students (Goe et al., 2008). Multicultural education theorists and scholars generally agree that in order for multicultural education interventions to be implemented successfully, institutional change toward inclusivity and equity must be made in the (a) curriculum, teaching materials, teaching and learning styles; (b) the attitudes, perceptions, and behaviors of teachers and administrators; and (c) the goals, norms, and culture of the school (Banks, 2001). Hence, we recommend that school leaders, educators, and SMH service providers engage in strategic discussions about feasible changes to be made in each of the three domains above to bolster culturally informed practices related to immigrant students. Specific changes may depend on each school and district, and some examples may include (a) infusing more content related to immigration, immigrants, and cultural diversity around the globe in curriculum and other educational material; (b) providing ongoing professional development opportunities to enhance teachers' culturally informed approaches by addressing attitudes, behaviors, and perceptions of immigrant students and their families (e.g., language discrimination, xenophobic attitudes, racist perceptions of students' ability); and (c) including immigrant students and families in conversations that are relevant to shaping the goals, norms, and culture of the school through parent-teaching meetings, leadership meetings, and town halls.

Importantly, teachers' ability to support students plays a role in their own psychological well-being, thus promoting less stress, burnout, and negative psychological symptoms among educators (Maslach & Leiter, 1999). Thus, embracing and providing culturally informed interventions aimed at supporting educators and administrators can be beneficial to everyone's well-being, including the students, their families, and the educators themselves. Mounting research is suggesting that culturally informed interventions help bolster the agency (e.g., perceived ability) of students and families, and reduce diversity-related burnout among educators (Cadenas et al., 2019; Cholewa et al., 2014; Crawford & Valle, 2016; Davidman & Davidman, 1997; Grayson & Alvarez, 2008; Guttentag et al., 2018, Xie et al., 2022). However, intervention and community-based research are needed to examine the best processes for providing such interventions to multiple audiences in the context of immigration in K-12 schools.

8.3.6 Multitiered Interventions for School Participation and Mental Health

Culturally informed Tier 1 interventions and programs that foster healthy relationships (peer, family, mentoring), safety, and a sense of belonging have been associated with positive well-being outcomes for immigrant youth (Arora et al., 2021; Marsh & Mathur, 2020). Gonzales et al. (2013) posited that opportunities for education, community participation, civic engagement, and belonging play a role in reducing anxiety. Creating further opportunities for connection within and outside of the classroom helps enhance positive relationships. Importantly, relationships between students and teachers have been found as key mediators for student's academic and social development (Suárez-Orozco et al., 2009). In addition, mentorship opportunities contribute to social-emotional-academic development and academic resilience of immigrant students (Gonzales, 2010; Portes & Fernandez-Kelly, 2008; Smith, 2008), highlighting the key role of supportive educators. Hence, the literature in this area suggests the importance of educators as Tier 1 intervenors to promote school participation.

Additionally, social support has been identified as a protective factor for immigrant students with a positive impact on identity formation, increased self-esteem, and feelings of empowerment that are key to consider in Tier 1 interventions (Garcini, et al., 2021). Cadenas et al. (2019) provided a summary of Tier 1 school-based interventions to promote the psychological well-being of immigrant youth, including undocumented youth and families, through an intersectional lens. These interventions included promoting intergroup contact and ally development among students and parents. This involves facilitating events that are inclusive to immigrant youth where the cultural identity of immigrants at the school can be celebrated. Furthermore, Tier 1 interventions also involve providing educational opportunities for parents and youth who are not immigrants to learn factual information about immigrants, and to learn how to be "allies" and supporters of immigrants. Finally, Tier 1 interventions should encourage activism and community engagement outlets for youth and families. This may involve supporting student-led or parent-led advocacy efforts to promote inclusivity of immigrants within the school, as well hosting events for parents to connect with local advocacy organizations, legal rights groups, and community leaders. These Tier 1 interventions are oriented toward promoting school participation by students and toward training school-based providers to becoming more welcoming so that immigrant youth and families can be comfortable with seeking services.

In addition to Tier 1 interventions, culturally informed and culturally adapted mental health evidence-based Tier 2 and 3 interventions are effective ways to support immigrant students in schools, including those who are undocumented (Arora et al., 2021). Tier 2 interventions, such as individual and group mental health support, can help students process their emotional experiences and gain coping skills to reduce distress related to immigration status. Support groups (e.g., process, educational, activity-based) have the added benefit of providing a sense of sameness and twinship (e.g., recognizing similarities with others who hold similar identities), experiences that contribute to an individual's sense of belonging (Kottler, 2015), feeling supported, and less alone. These groups may be offered specifically to immigrant students based on aspects of their identity. Furthermore, it is important to consider supporting the professional development of SMH providers to offer specialized Tier 3 interventions to immigrant youth. This may include providing specialized training to school counselors and SMH providers, particularly training to develop competencies in providing services to promote effective SMH while integrating cultural humility and sensitivity to systemic stressors (e.g., anti-immigrant policies), as well as clinical interventions to address trauma with minoritized groups (Cadenas et al., 2019).

8.4 ImmSchools: Creating Safe and Welcoming Schools for Undocumented Youth

ImmSchools is a culmination of the life, work, and everyday experiences of its founders, who grew up undocumented in the K-12 education system. In 2017, Viridiana Carrizales enlisted the support of Vanessa Luna and Lorena Tule-Romain to form ImmSchools and support educators in creating the kinds of supportive schools they and their families wished they had. ImmSchools founding team is composed of formerly undocumented immigrant women with a combined 15+ years working in the intersection of education and immigration. ImmSchools' mission is to create safe and welcoming schools for the 4.9 million K-12 students who are either undocumented or living in a "mixed status" household with at least one undocumented immigrant parent (Connor, 2021). ImmSchools carries out their mission by partnering with K-12 educators, school districts, community leaders, and students and families across the nation. ImmSchools provides the entire school community—including students and families themselves along with their teachers and administrators—with programs and resources to build safe and welcoming environments for undocumented students and those from mixed-status families.

Prior to launching ImmSchools as a national nonprofit, the founders interviewed dozens of immigrant families and students, educators, and community leaders to learn about their needs and their recommendations for creating more equitable educational opportunities. After an initial pilot in 2018 in San Antonio, Texas, ImmSchools expanded into New York City the same year, and later to Dallas, Texas, and Camden, New Jersey. ImmSchools continues to operate in these four locations and will continue to deepen its reach in these three states over the next several years in response to significant need: more than 25% of the country's undocumented families and 10% of all K-12 students living in mixed-status families live in these three states. A key component of ImmSchools approach is that its team is composed of currently or formerly undocumented immigrants, individuals who grew up in mixed-status or immigrant families. This lived experience centers the expertise of proximate and directly impacted individuals to bring forward transformational change in our schools.

While ImmSchools was not designed as a program to address SMH through direct clinical intervention services, its approach to facilitating educational empowerment of immigrant youth, families, and educators can be conceptualized as a Tier 1 intervention (Arora et al., 2021; Marsh & Mathur, 2020). The educational intervention programs aim to address multiple factors that contribute to shifting school culture to become safer and more welcoming toward immigrants and undocumented youth. By focusing their interventions at the structural level, ImmSchools seeks to promote the overall well-being of immigrants in school contexts. Since its launch, ImmSchools has trained more than 10,000 educators in 30+ districts and schools and reached more than 3300 students and 4900 parents through workshops in areas with some of the highest proportions of immigrant residents: New York City; Dallas Fort Worth and San Antonio, Texas; and Camden, New Jersey. More than 90% of educator participants indicate that they are better able to support immigrant students, and 97% of students and family participants say they have greater access to resources and knowledge on immigration and education.

8.4.1   The Theory of Change

Schools have the responsibility to ensure all students, regardless of immigration status, feel safe and welcome. However, as a result of the silence around and misinformation about the topic of immigration in our schools, this is far from the reality for the undocumented community. Currently, school districts are unaware how to enact pro-immigrant policies, educators are unaware of how to create inclusive curricula, families are unaware of how to engage with educators, and students are unaware of available resources (Amuedo-Dorantes et al., 2022; Cadenas et al., 2021; Cadenas et al., 2019; Cha et al., 2019; Constantine & Gushue, 2003). This lack of awareness can lead to fear and uncertainty for students that meaningfully impact their educational engagement, well-being, and academic performance. Moreover, undocumented students face countless psychological stressors such as the constant fear of immigration enforcement and deportation, economic insecurity, and language barriers that affect their ability to thrive in school (Ee & Gándara, 2020a, b). Due to immigration enforcement alone, a Harvard Policy Brief revealed that 85% students expressed fears while at school, 79.6% experienced increased behavioral and/or emotional problems, and 64.7% indirect effects on the school climate (Ee & Gándara, 2020a, b). In a national survey conducted by UCLA Civil Rights Project (Gándara & Ee, 2018), 84% of 5400 educators interviewed noted that their students expressed concerns about immigration enforcement issues at school. Ultimately, these pressures can drastically impair a child's sense of safety, socio-emotional well-being, and academic performance in K-12. Moreover, children can only experience deep learning if they are cognitively and emotionally engaged with the content before them, which is dependent on interacting in a safe space (Romero, 2015).

ImmSchools' theory of change (ImmSchools, 2022; see Fig. 8.1) is centered on transforming schools into safe and welcoming spaces by partnering with educators and community leaders to provide tailored interventions that shift school culture and center the experiences of undocumented students in order for them to thrive and reach their fullest potential. ImmSchools directly targets immigrant-dense schools that are ready for and committed to change and, by providing district/school leaders and other constituents in those schools (educators, students, and families) with focused, tailored support each year based on their needs, supports partner schools to develop a safe and welcoming school culture plan around these focus areas: (1) administrative action, (2) educator preparedness, (3) engagement, empowerment, and advocacy among students and families (Fig. 8.1).

Through the development of a rubric built with student and family input, ImmSchools measures the process of each individual school partner in shifting school culture. ImmSchools' Welcoming School Culture Rubric defines a safe and welcoming school culture as one in which administrators implement pro-immigrant policies; educators employ culturally informed practices and anti-racist curricula; and students and families increase participation in school and community spaces, as well as leverage educational and legal resources. Each dimension is scored on a 3-point scale each year. At the end of each year, ImmSchools aims for partner schools to see a 1-point increase in at least 1 dimension. The goal is that over the course of a 2–3 year partnership, schools will score at least a 2 out of 3 on all dimensions of the rubric. In the past year from June 2022 through May 2023, ImmSchools implemented this rubric evaluation and scoring process with 14 multiyear partnerships. At the end of the fiscal year, 92% of school partners increased by at least 0.5 points and 79% increased by at least 1 point on the 3-point rubric scale in their selected focus area as a direct result of ImmSchools' programs and consulting.

One case study that particularly illuminates how the rubric operationalizes and measures ImmSchools' impact in a specific focus area includes a school in a predominantly Black, Indigenous, and other People of Color (BIPOC) immigrant

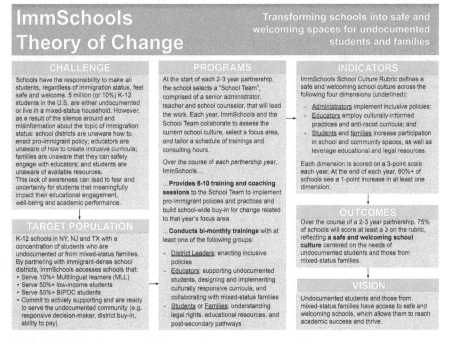

Fig. 8.1 ImmSchools theory of change

community located in New York City, which we would refer to as School A. This school chose to focus on the "Student Engagement" set of educational interventions for their first year of the multiyear partnership. As a part of the "Student Engagement" focus area, the rubric tracks the school's progress with increasing students' participation, agency, and access. For example, a score of a "1" or underdeveloped under students' agency can be observed as students provided with little to no opportunity to occupy school and district leadership positions, while a score of a "3" or developed can be observed as students occupying school and district leadership positions at the same rate as their peers.

Over the course of the year, ImmSchools hosted multiple student workshops and family meetings co-led with students at School A that deliberately carved a safe space to discuss immigrant rights, college access as an undocumented student, anti-bullying tools, and mental health resources. These workshops aimed to specifically build undocumented and immigrant students' participation, agency, and access under the "Student Engagement" focus area. By the end of the first year, School A's BIPOC immigrant students launched a Multicultural Club with elected student leaders as part of its Dream Squad efforts which clearly and powerfully promoted student's participation in that they occupied leadership positions. "Regardless of who we are, we still have the opportunities to fulfill our dreams," noted one student participant.

As part of the second year of ImmSchools' multiyear partnership, School A has chosen our "Administrative Action" focus area. Through this focus area, ImmSchools has hosted four professional development sessions for School A's chosen School Team members, four professional development sessions for their school staff, and three coaching/consulting hours. As a result of these interventions, school staff and administration have updated enrollment procedures to actively support undocumented and mixed-status enrollment. In accordance with our Inclusive School Culture Rubric, ImmSchools' programs have propelled School A's "Administrative Action" scoring by 1.5 points.

8.4.2 ImmSchools: School-Based Interventions

ImmSchools aims to increase school participation, increase use of educational resources, improve school culture, and improve psychological well-being among youth and families. The educational intervention programs provided by ImmSchools are informed by personal experiences of undocumented students and families, by experiences of educators who serve this community, as well as by extant research. These programs are delivered in partnership with K-12 schools in four metropolitan areas across three states (New York, New Jersey, and Texas), and are implemented as three programmatic pillars designed for specific populations: (1) responding to the needs of undocumented youth and families through programs for empowerment and school engagement, (2) preparing educators to engage in culturally informed practiced with immigrants students, and (3) supporting administrators to develop plans to shift practices and policies at the school level (ImmSchools, 2022). These target groups receive a range of intervention programs, including specialized trainings for educators (as a set of three sessions lasting 90 min), individual workshops for students and parents, and coaching sessions for administrators (e.g., facilitated dialogues for critical reflection). Topics included in programming for youth and families are legal and educational resources, "know your rights" legal education, eligibility for college and scholarships, and school engagement. In addition, ImmSchools programs elevate students and family leadership by developing multi-generational interventions which are co-facilitated or directly led by undocumented students and families. Undocumented students and family members are provided opportunities to lead spaces within schools and classrooms, and they are centered in the planning and execution of programs for transforming school culture.

Transforming the culture in schools to become safer and more welcoming to undocumented youth and families involves providing support to school educators and administrators. Thus, ImmSchools aims to support school educators and administrators in the implementation of welcoming policies, helps prepare them to make use of culturally informed practices and anti-racist curriculum, and promote their psychological well-being. Topics covered in programming for educators and administrators include culturally responsive pedagogy, creating a safe school environment and mental health of immigrant children and families, enacting and implementing pro-immigrant school policies, and developing and implementing a "Safe & Welcoming School Plan."

To implement this programming, ImmSchools staff collaborate with a School Team, which includes a diverse group of school staff such as administrator, school leader, teacher, school counselor, and other supporting staff in each school. These school teams are assembled by the partner school in collaboration with ImmSchools staff, and may draw from existing school-based teams (e.g., social, emotional behavioral, and mental health [SEBMH] lead team) that support students and families. In order to focus their efforts and choose schools to partner with, ImmSchools prioritizes serving schools that meet two of the following criteria: (1) Over 10% of students are English Language Learners. (2) Over 50% of students come from low-income backgrounds. (3) Over 50% of the students are BIPOC, including Latinx and Asian. (4) Schools commit to actively supporting and serving undocumented students. ImmSchools programs aim to promote the educational empowerment of youth, families, and educators supporting them to shift school culture toward immigrant and undocumented students. The goal is that the overall well-being of immigrants and the educators supporting them can be enhanced by focusing on helping schools become safer and more welcoming toward immigrants. The programs are offered broadly to all students to prevent the segregation of immigrant and undocumented students, further excluding them. By providing the programs to all students at the school, those students who are not immigrants and undocumented may also learn about resources to support their peers and may also benefit from culturally affirming interventions.

8.4.3   Assessing Impact and Promoting Change Through Participatory Action Research (PAR)

The intervention programs provided by ImmSchools are already having a tangible impact, reaching about 12,000 students, families, school educators, and administrators. Presently, ImmSchools is engaged in a multiyear project that blends Participatory Action Research (PAR; Baum et al., 2006) and quantitative methodologies designed to gather evidence regarding the effectiveness of educational intervention programs aspiring to transform the culture in schools. The study holds approval by a university's Institutional Review Board (IRB). The central research question is: What are the immediate effects of ImmSchools programs on undocumented youth, undocumented families, educators, and school leaders?

This project used PAR methods to enhance an assessment tool to capture ImmSchools' impact targeting three populations receiving services (undocumented youth and families, educators, education leaders) across three states varying in welcoming policies (i.e., New York, New Jersey, and Texas). The assessment tool was enhanced by infusing psychometrically sound measures that were reviewed and chosen collaboratively by the Community Research Team, which is made up of first- and second-generation immigrants of color who work as staff at ImmSchools or who are researchers (i.e., faculty and graduate students) at a major research university in the Northeast of the United States. The new assessment tool includes validated measures of psychological well-being of students, families, and educators. Furthermore, measures for students and parents include measures of school participation, social self-efficacy, and school culture. Measures for educators include assessments of culturally informed practices with undocumented student and school culture. Data are being collected during ImmSchools programs, including pre- and post-program assessments, as well as follow-up assessments 6-months and 1-year after the programs conclude. The researchers are conducting quantitative and qualitative analysis to probe research questions. These analyses are being conducted and interpreted using a PAR framework. This means that the researchers engage in ongoing dialogue about how quantitative findings reflect and align with the lived experiences of immigrant youth, families, and educators.

Consistent with PAR methodologies, this research project uses critical self-reflection and collaboration as central tools in its implementation. This includes dedicating time in each research meeting to discuss the researchers' positionality and culture, experiences with racism and anti-racism, and to process recent changes to immigration policy (e.g., courts' rulings on the Deferred Action for Childhood Arrivals program). As far assessment, the research team examined the existing survey developed by ImmSchools leaders and suggested additional validated measures to be integrated in the survey, and considered questions and measures developed by school districts and departments of education. We have continued to thoughtfully consider research procedures (e.g., streamlined data collection, minimizing risk in data storage), prioritizing translation of surveys into several languages to increase accessibility, providing research training focused on PAR and anti-racism to ImmSchools program facilitators, and discussing and resisting ethno-racial hierarchies within the research and publication process. This research process has been enriched by PAR methodologies that center the experiences of undocumented students and families in all aspects of it.

Additionally, the project aims to implement advocacy efforts that are informed by research findings. The hope is for this action research to support the transformation of practice and policy to widely adopt educational interventions that are effective in reducing inequalities that disadvantage undocumented youth. This advocacy is to be guided by a Community Advisory Board (CAB), which is also composed of eight immigrants of color, including current and formerly undocumented immigrants, who have expertise at the intersection of education and immigration. These advocacy efforts may include launching a public report with findings and recommendations for best practices, as well as bringing findings from the research to policymakers and educational practitioners. Findings from this research will also be shared in academic outlets to inform future research, with educational practitioners to inform school practices, and will be used for advocacy with policymakers at the school, district, state, and national levels. Assessments for this research project were launched in the fall, 2022, preliminary data analysis took place in 2023, findings from the project are being shared publicly and in academic outlets in 2024, and once publicly available, ImmSchools leaders and community members may leverage these preliminary findings for advocacy within schools, districts, departments of education, and state-level policymakers.

Preliminary findings from the first year of the project are beginning to emerge based on survey assessments from the 2022–2023 school year. A total of 91 students, 71 family members, and 57 educators completed program surveys after participating in the Tier 1 intervention programs offered by ImmSchools. Preliminary findings from quantitative data analysis suggest that students and families reported greater psychological well-being at the end of the program. For students, there were associations between psychological well-being, welcoming school climate, positive academic engagement, and self-efficacy for obtaining support from parents and teachers. Preliminary findings from parents suggested that after the program, parents tended to experience schools as having an inclusive school culture and that this was associated with feeling welcomed at the school. Additionally, there were associations between inclusive school culture, school participation, and psychological well-being for parents. Finally, themes from the analysis suggest that educators tended to feel more informed and competent to teach immigrant students after the programs. These early findings are beginning to highlight the relationship between context (i.e., welcoming school, school culture) and several positive outcomes (e.g., psychological well-being) among students, parents, and educators who participated in ImmSchools Tier 1 programs.

8.5 Conclusion

Students of color who come from minoritized racial and ethnic groups are projected to become the majority of students in K-12 schools in the United States in the near future. This includes a sizeable number of immigrant students, including those who are undocumented or who live in mixed-status families. This chapter reviewed the research establishing the connection between school-level experiences (e.g., school participation, culturally informed practices) and the mental health of undocumented youth, their families, and the educators that serve them. Responding to the dearth of literature pertaining to interventions to support immigrant students in schools, this chapter described the intervention approach by ImmSchools. This immigrant-led nonprofit organization aims to contribute to solutions and promising practices in support of undocumented students and families in K-12 schools, and to ultimately promote their well-being. This chapter also described a Participatory Action Research (PAR) project that is underway to assess the positive impact of ImmSchools programs, and to leverage this evidence to inform educational policy and practice. We hope that this chapter will be of use to researchers, educators, and policymakers in exploring how to reach traditionally underserved populations, such as undocumented students and their families.

References

Abrego, L. J. (2011). Legal consciousness of undocumented Latinos: Fear and stigma as barriers to claims-making for first-and 1.5-generation immigrants. *Law & Society Review, 45*(2), 337–370.

Amuedo-Dorantes, C., Bucheli, J. R., & Martinez-Donate, A. P. (2022). Safe-zone schools and children with undocumented parents. In *Parent-child separation* (pp. 3–28). Springer.

Arora, P. G., Alvarez, K., Huang, C., & Wang, C. (2021). A three-tiered model for addressing the mental health needs of immigrant-origin youth in schools. *Journal of Immigrant and Minority Health, 23*(1), 151–162. https://doi.org/10.1007/s10903-020-01048-9

Bandura, A. (2006). Guide for constructing self-efficacy scales. In F. Pajares & T. Urdan (Eds.), *Self-efficacy beliefs of adolescents* (Vol. 5, pp. 307–337). Information Age Publishing.

Banks, J. A. (1989). Multicultural education: Characteristics and goals. In J. Banks & C. Banks (Eds.), *Multicultural education: Issues and perspectives*. Allyn and Bacon.

Banks, J. A. (1993). Multicultural education: Historical development, dimensions, and practice. *Review of Research in Education, 19*, 3–49. https://doi.org/10.2307/1167339

Banks, J. A. (2001). Multicultural education: Historical development, dimensions, and practice. In J. A. Banks & C. A. McGee Banks (Eds.), *Handbook of research on multicultural education* (pp. 3–24). Jossey Bass, Inc.

Baum, F., MacDougall, C., & Smith, D. (2006). Participatory action research. *Journal of Epidemiology and Community Health, 60*(10), 854. https://doi.org/10.1136/jech.2004.028662

Cadenas, G. A., Cisneros, J., Todd, N. R., & Spanierman, L. B. (2018). DREAMzone: Testing two vicarious contact interventions to improve attitudes toward undocumented immigrants. *Journal of Diversity in Higher Education, 11*(3), 295.

Cadenas, G., Peña, D., & Cisneros, J. (2019). Creating a welcoming environment of mental health equity for undocumented students. In *Educational leadership of immigrants* (pp. 71–78). Routledge.

Cadenas, G. A., Cisneros, J., Spanierman, L. B., Yi, J., & Todd, N. R. (2021). Detrimental effects of color-blind racial attitudes in preparing a culturally responsive teaching workforce for immigrants. *Journal of Career Development, 48*(6), 926–941. https://doi.org/10.1177/0894845320903380

Cadenas, G. A., Cerezo, A., Carlos Chavez, F. L., Capielo Rosario, C., Torres, L., Suro, B., Fuentes, M., & Sanchez, D. (2022). The citizenship shield: Mediated and moderated links between immigration status, discrimination, food insecurity, and negative health outcomes for latinx immigrants during the COVID-19 pandemic. *Journal of Community Psychology*. https://doi.org/10.1002/jcop.22831. Advance online publication.

Capps, R., Fix, M., & Zong, J. (2016). *A profile of US children with unauthorized immigrant parents*. Migration Policy Institute.

Cavazos-Rehg, P. A., Zayas, L. H., & Spitznagel, E. L. (2007). Legal status, emotional well-being and subjective health status of Latino immigrants. *Journal of the National Medical Association, 99*(10), 1126.

Cha, B. S., Enriquez, L. E., & Ro, A. (2019). Beyond access: Psychosocial barriers to undocumented students' use of mental health services. *Social Science & Medicine, 1982*(233), 193–200. https://doi.org/10.1016/j.socscimed.2019.06.003

Chan, K. S. (2001). US-born, immigrant, refugee, or indigenous status: public policy implications for Asian Pacific American families. See Chang, 2001, 197–229.

Cheng, Y. Y. (2012). *Re-conceptualizing parentified children from immigrant families*. Alliant International University.

Cholewa, B., Goodman, R., West-Olatunji, C., & Amatea, E. (2014). A 1ualitative examination of the impact of culturally responsive educational practices on the psychological well-being of students of color. *The Urban Review, 46*, 574. https://doi.org/10.1007/s11256-014-0272-y

Cisneros, J., & Cadenas, G. (2017). DREAMer-ally competency and self-efficacy: Developing higher education staff and measuring lasting outcomes. *Journal of Student Affairs Research and Practice, 54*(2), 189–203. https://doi.org/10.1080/19496591.2017.1289098

Coll, C. G., & Marks, A. K. (2012). *The immigrant paradox in children and adolescents: Is becoming American a developmental risk?* American Psychological Association. https://doi.org/10.1037/13094-000

Coll, C. G., Patton, F., Marks, A. K., Dimitrova, R., Yang, R., Suarez, G. A., & Patrico, A. (2012). Understanding the immigrant paradox in youth: Developmental and contextual considerations. In A. S. Masten, K. Liebkind, & D. J. Hernandez (Eds.), *Realizing the potential of immigrant youth* (pp. 159–180). Cambridge University Press. https://doi.org/10.1017/CBO9781139094696.009

Connor, P. (2021). *Immigration reform can keep millions of mixed-status families together.* Retrieved from https://www.fwd.us/news/mixed-status-families/

Constantine, M. G., & Gushue, G. V. (2003). School counselors' ethnic tolerance attitudes and racism attitudes as predictors of their multicultural case conceptualization of an immigrant student. *Journal of Counseling & Development, 81*(2), 185–190.

Crawford, E. R., & Dorner, L. M. (Eds.). (2019). Educational leadership of immigrants: Case studies in times of change. Routledge.

Crawford, E. R., & Valle, F. (2016). Educational justice for undocumented students: How school counselors encourage student persistence in schools. *Education Policy Analysis Archives, 24*(98), 10.14507/epaa.24.242.

Crosnoe, R., & Turley, R. N. (2011). K-12 educational outcomes of immigrant youth. *The Future of Children, 21*(1), 129–152. https://doi.org/10.1353/foc.2011.0008

Davidman, L., & Davidman, P. (1997). *Teaching with a multicultural perspective: A practical guide.* Longman.

Diaz, Y., & Fenning, P. (2021). Toward understanding mental health concerns for the Latinx immigrant student: A review of the literature. *Urban Education, 56*(6), 959–981.

Ee, J., & Gándara, P. (2020a). The impact of immigration enforcement on the nation's schools. *American Educational Research Journal, 57*(2), 840–871. https://doi.org/10.3102/0002831219862998

Ee, J., & Gándara, P. (2020b). *Under siege: The disturbing impact of immigration enforcement on the nation's schools* (Immigration initiative at Harvard issue brief series no. 2). Harvard University.

Fix, M., & Zimmermann, W. (2001). All under one roof: Mixed-status families in an era of reform 1. *International Migration Review, 35*(2), 397–419.

Gándara, P., & Ee, J. (2018). *U.S. immigration enforcement policy and its impact on teaching and learning in the nation's schools.* The Civil Rights Project-Proyecto Derechos Civiles at UCLA.

Garcini, L. M., Daly, R., Chen, N., Mehl, J., Pham, T., Phan, T., Hansen, B., & Kothare, A. (2021). Undocumented immigrants and mental health: A systematic review of recent methodology and findings in the U.S. *Journal of Migration and Health, 4*, 100058. https://doi.org/10.1016/j.jmh.2021.100058

Gay, G. (2004). Curriculum theory and multicultural education. In J. Banks (Ed.), *Handbook of research on multicultural education* (2nd ed., pp. 30–49). Jossey-Bass.

Gay, G. (2010a). *Culturally responsive teaching theory, research, and practice* (2nd ed.). Teachers College Press.

Gay, G. (2010b). Teaching literacy in cultural context. In K. Dunsmore & D. Douglas (Eds.), *Bringing literacy home* (pp. 161–183). International Reading Association. https://doi.org/10.1598/0711.07

Goe, L., Bell, C., & Little, O. (2008). *Approaches to evaluating teacher effectiveness: A research synthesis.* Retrieved from ERIC database. (ED521228).

Gonzales, R. G. (2010). On the wrong side of the tracks: Understanding the effects of school structure and social capital in the educational pursuits of undocumented immigrant students. *Peabody Journal of Education, 85*(4), 469–485.

Gonzales, R. G. (2016). Lives in limbo: Undocumented and coming of age in America. Univ of California Press.

Gonzales, R. G., & Chavez, L. R. (2012). Awakening to a nightmare abjectivity and illegality in the lives of undocumented 1.5-generation Latino immigrants in the United States. *Current Anthropology, 53*(3), 255–281.

Gonzales, R. G., & Ruiz, A. G. (2014). Dreaming beyond the fields: Undocumented youth, rural realities and a constellation of disadvantage. *Latino Studies, 12*, 194–216.

Gonzales, R. G., Suárez-Orozco, C., & Dedios-Sanguineti, M. C. (2013). No place to belong: Contextualizing concepts of mental health among undocumented immigrant youth in the U.S. *American Behavioral Scientist, 57*(8), 1174–1199. https://doi.org/10.1177/0002764213487349

Grayson, J., & Alvarez, H. K. (2008). School climate factors relating to teacher burnout: A mediator model, teaching and teacher education. *International Journal of Research Studies, 24*(5), 1349–1363, ISSN 0742-051X. https://doi.org/10.1016/j.tate.2007.06.005

Gutentag, T., Horenczyk, G., & Tatar, M. (2018). Teachers' approaches toward cultural diversity predict diversity-related burnout and self-efficacy. *Journal of Teacher Education, 69*(4), 408–419. https://doi.org/10.1177/0022487117714244

Hernandez, S., Hernandez, I., Jr., Gadson, R., Huftalin, D., Ortiz, A. M., White, M. C., & Yocum-Gaffney, D. (2010). Sharing their secrets: Undocumented students' personal stories of fear, drive, and survival. *New Directions for Student Services, 2010*(131), 67–84.

ImmSchools. (2022). *Theory of change: Transforming schools into safe and welcoming spaces for undocumented students and families.* ImmSchools.

Jefferies, J., & Dabach, D. B. (2014). Breaking the silence: Facing undocumented issues in teacher practice. *Association of Mexican American Educators Journal, 8*(1).

John-Akinola, Y. O., & Nic-Gabhainn, S. (2014). Children's participation in school: A cross-sectional study of the relationship between school environments, participation and health and well-being outcomes. *BMC Public Health, 14*(1), 1–10.

Kemmak, A. R., Nargesi, S., & Saniee, N. (2021). Social determinant of mental health in immigrants and refugees: A systematic review. *Medical Journal of the Islamic Republic of Iran, 35*, 196.

Korpershoek, H., King, R. B., McInerney, D. M., Nasser, R. N., Ganotice, F. A., & Watkins, D. A. (2021). Gender and cultural differences in school motivation. *Research Papers in Education, 36*(1), 27–51.

Kottler, A. (2015). Feeling at home, belonging, and being human: Kohut, self psychology, twinship, and alienation. *International Journal of Psychoanalytic Self Psychology, 10*(4), 378–389.

Lad, K., & Braganza, D. (2013). Increasing knowledge related to the experiences of undocumented immigrants in public schools. *Educational Leadership and Administration: Teaching and Program Development, 24*, 1–15.

Marsh, R. J., & Mathur, S. R. (2020). Mental health in schools: An overview of multi-tiered systems of support. *Intervention in School and Clinic, 56*(2), 67–73. https://doi.org/10.1177/1053451220914896

Maslach, C., & Leiter, M. P. (1999). Teacher burnout: A research agenda. In R. Vandenberghe & A. M. Huberman (Eds.), *Understanding and preventing teacher burnout: A sourcebook of international research and practice* (pp. 295–303). Cambridge University Press. https://doi.org/10.1017/CBO9780511527784.021

Metzner, F., Adedeji, A., Wichmann, M. L. Y., Zaheer, Z., Schneider, L., Schlachzig, L., Richters, J., Heumann, S., & Mays, D. (2022). Experiences of discrimination and everyday racism among children and adolescents with an immigrant background–Results of a systematic literature review on the impact of discrimination on the developmental outcomes of minors worldwide. *Frontiers in Psychology, 13*, 805941.

Motti-Stefanidi, F., & Masten, A. S. (2013). School success and school engagement of immigrant children and adolescents. European Psychologist.

Nienhusser, H. K. (2013). Role of High Schools in Undocumented Students' College Choice. *Education Policy Analysis Archives, 21*(85), n85.

Parkhouse, H., Massaro, V., Cuba, M. J., & Waters, C. N. (2020). Teachers' efforts to support undocumented students within ambiguous policy contexts. *Harvard Educational Review, 90*, 525.

Portes, A., & Fernández-Kelly, P. (2008). No margin for error: Educational and occupational achievement among disadvantaged children of immigrants. *The Annals of the American Academy of Political and Social Science, 620*(1), 12–36.

Qin, K., Colomer, S. E., Yu, L., & Cole, C. (2022). Negotiating racialized discourses and navigating racism in US schools: Understanding Chinese immigrants' parenting identities and practices through an AsianCrit lens. *Urban Education.* https://doi.org/10.1177/00420859221089551

Romero, C. (2015). *What we know about belonging from scientific research.* Mindset Scholars Network, Center for Advanced Study in the Behavioral Sciences, Stanford University. Retrieved from http://mindsetscholarsnetwork.org/wp-content/uploads/2015/09/What-We-Know-About-Belonging.pdf

Sidhu, S. S. (2017). Impact of recent executive actions on minority youth and families. *Journal of the American Academy of Child and Adolescent Psychiatry, 56*(10), 805–807. https://doi.org/10.1016/j.jaac.2017.07.779

Sigona, N., Gonzales, R. G., Franco, M. C., & Papoutsi, A. (2019). *Undocumented migration.* Wiley.

Smith, R. C. (2008). Horatio Alger lives in Brooklyn: Extrafamily support, intrafamily dynamics, and socially neutral operating identities in exceptional mobility among children of Mexican immigrants. *The Annals of the American Academy of Political and Social Science, 620*(1), 270–290.

Suárez-Orozco, C., Rhodes, J., & Milburn, M. (2009). Unraveling the immigrant paradox: Academic engagement and disengagement among recently arrived immigrant youth. *Youth & Society, 41*(2), 151–185.

Suárez-Orozco, C., Yoshikawa, H., & Tseng, V. (2015). *Intersecting inequalities: Research to reduce inequality for immigrant-origin children and youth.* William T. Grant Foundation.

Todd, A., Ayala, C., & Barraza, K. (2020). School counselors working with undocumented students in k-12 school settings. *Journal of School Counseling, 18*(14), n14.

Torres-Olave, B. M., Torrez, M. A., Ferguson, K., Bedford, A., Castillo-Lavergne, C. M., Robles, K., & Chang, A. (2021). Fuera de lugar: Undocumented students, dislocation, and the search for belonging. *Journal of Diversity in Higher Education, 14*(3), 418.

U.S. Census Bureau. (2019). *Census Bureau reports nearly 77 million students enrolled in U.S. Schools.* https://www.census.gov/newsroom/press-releases/2011ed/in/U.S./Schools

Xie, M., Huang, S., Ke, L., Wang, X., & Wang, Y. (2022). The development of teacher burnout and the effects of resource factors: A latent transition perspective. *International Journal of Environmental Research and Public Health, 19*(5), 2725. https://doi.org/10.3390/ijerph19052725

Zong, J., & Batalova, J. (2019). *How many unauthorized immigrants graduate from U.S. high schools annually?* Migration Policy Institute. https://www.migrationpolicy.org/research/unauthorized-immigrants-graduate-us-high-schools

Index

Printed in the USA
CPSIA information can be obtained
at www.ICGtesting.com
CBHW050236211024
16148CB00004B/224

9 783031 681677